DK American College
of Physicians

PROSTATE
PROBLEMS

D1412036

DISCARD

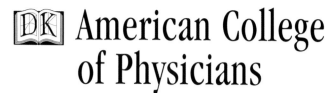

American College of Physicians

HOME MEDICAL GUIDE *to*

PROSTATE
PROBLEMS

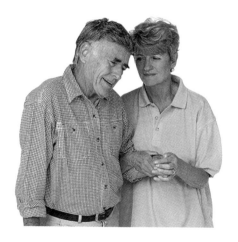

MEDICAL EDITOR
DAVID R. GOLDMANN, MD
ASSOCIATE MEDICAL EDITOR
DAVID A. HOROWITZ, MD

A DORLING KINDERSLEY BOOK

IMPORTANT

The American College of Physicians (ACP) Home Medical Guides provide general information on a wide range of health and medical topics. These books are not substitutes for medical diagnosis, and you should always consult your doctor on personal health matters before undertaking any program of therapy or treatment. Various medical organizations have different guidelines for diagnosis and treatment of the same conditions; the American College of Physicians–American Society of Internal Medicine (ACP–ASIM) has tried to present a reasonable consensus of these opinions.

Material in this book was reviewed by the ACP–ASIM for general medical accuracy and applicability in the United States; however, the information provided herein does not necessarily reflect the specific recommendations or opinions of the ACP–ASIM. The naming of any organization, product, or alternative therapy in these books is not an ACP–ASIM endorsement, and the omission of any such name does not indicate ACP–ASIM disapproval.

DORLING KINDERSLEY
LONDON, NEW YORK, AUCKLAND, DELHI, JOHANNESBURG, MUNICH, PARIS, AND SYDNEY

DK www.dk.com

Senior Editors Jill Hamilton, Nicki Lampon
Senior Designer Jan English
DTP Design Jason Little
Editor Nicholas Mulcahy
Medical Consultant Eric S. Rovner, MD

Senior Managing Editor Martyn Page
Senior Managing Art Editor Bryn Walls

Published in the United States in 2000 by
Dorling Kindersley Publishing, Inc.,
95 Madison Avenue, New York, New York 10016

2 4 6 8 10 9 7 5 3 1

Library of Congress Catalog Card Number 99-76853
ISBN 0-7894-4178-3

Reproduced by Colourscan, Singapore
Printed and bound in the United States by Quebecor World, Taunton, Massachusetts

Contents

INTRODUCTION 7

THE PROSTATE AND ITS PROBLEMS 10

OTHER CONDITIONS CAUSING
"PROSTATE SYMPTOMS" 22

INVESTIGATING THE PROSTATE 27

HOW IS BPH TREATED? 37

URINARY RETENTION 50

PROSTATE-SPECIFIC ANTIGEN 53

PROSTATE CANCER 58

PROSTATITIS 75

IMPROVING TREATMENT 78

CASE HISTORIES 83

QUESTIONS AND ANSWERS 88

USEFUL ADDRESSES 91

NOTES 92

INDEX 94

ACKNOWLEDGMENTS 96

Introduction

Men often have difficulty addressing illness and debilitation, especially when it involves urinary or sexual function.

Prostate disorders have been a ready source of humor for comedians' barbs and TV situation comedies for years. However, although prostate disease may have been a source of popular amusement, it has not really been something for polite conversation and has rarely been discussed openly and seriously. The symptoms that are produced by various prostate disorders can be embarrassing.

Men too often feel that illness, particularly one involving the part of the body around the prostate, is degrading and is therefore something to be ashamed of. Moreover, since prostate symptoms are so common that most men have friends who are similarly affected, they view the problems as an inevitable and incurable part of growing old. In recent years, however, there has been a change in attitude of the public, the media, and many doctors to this very common problem. Now, almost every newspaper and magazine prints articles on the prostate. Famous people who have had prostate trouble are even interviewed about their experiences.

THE POTENTIAL PATIENT
Prostate problems of various kinds are common among all men. No one should feel embarrassed to discuss the symptoms of prostate disorders with his doctor.

7

The publicity surrounding the prostate cancer of celebrities such as former Presidential candidate Bob Dole and New York Yankees manager Joe Torre reminds us that prostate disease is a common problem in men. In 1997, a medical correspondent of a major daily paper underwent surgery for prostate cancer and wrote about his experiences.

New tests are available for the early diagnosis of prostate cancer. There are "Prostate Cancer Awareness Weeks," and many more men now have surgery to cure early prostate cancer. Fortunately, in most men, prostatic symptoms do not necessarily indicate life-threatening cancer. Symptoms are usually those of a benign condition, and treatment can usually improve quality of life. However, because of the increased awareness of prostate cancer, prostate disorders now have become an unnecessary cause of concern for many men.

Until recently, all that could be done for the most common form of prostate disease was an operation. This frightened many men and was one of the reasons for neglecting symptoms in the past. Now, there are new treatments and they have been well publicized. This publicity has made many men, perhaps previously afraid of what might happen to them, seek help. However, it also raised expectations too high, and there has been some disappointment. For many men, an operation is still the best solution.

This book explains diseases of the prostate, how they cause problems, and what can be done about them.

KEY POINTS

- Men with prostate symptoms should not feel embarrassed about discussing their problem with their doctor.
- New treatments for prostate problems are available to improve the quality of life.

The prostate and its problems

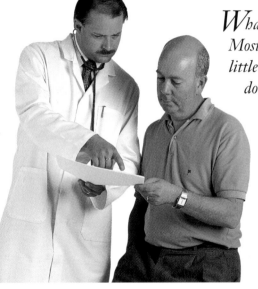

What is the prostate anyway? Most people have heard of it but have little idea of its purpose. Many people do not even know its location. Indeed, doctors and scientists do not fully understand the prostate's functions. There is still a lot to be learned about the prostate and the diseases that affect it.

A SIGN OF AGE
The prostate of most men becomes larger, particularly after the age of 50. When the enlargement affects urination, it is time to consult a doctor.

The prostate gland is located just underneath the bladder. It makes a portion of the seminal fluid released at the climax of the sexual act. The prostate needs hormones from the testes to function properly. If the levels of these male hormones are low, the prostate shrinks.

The fluid from glands is made in the epithelium, in layers of special cells called epithelial cells. In all glands, the epithelium is surrounded by tissue called stroma. In the prostate, this stroma contains muscle fibers that affect its function. Both the epithelium and the stroma increase in size if the prostate enlarges.

The Position of the Prostate Gland

The prostate gland lies beneath the bladder, and the urethra (carrying urine from the bladder to the opening of the penis) passes through it. The two tubes carrying semen and seminal fluid (the vas deferens) join the urethra inside the prostate.

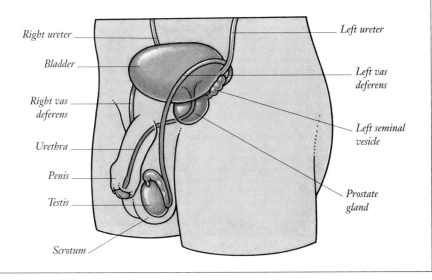

In addition, although the prostate looks like a single organ, it really has two different parts, each of which is prone to different diseases.

The prostate consists of an inner and an outer part (see p.12), both of which are made up of glands (epithelium) surrounded by tissue (stroma) containing muscle. Close to the prostate are two important muscles called sphincters. These muscles prevent the leakage of urine from the bladder. They also prevent the sperm and seminal fluid from entering the bladder during the climax of the sexual act. The muscle located below the prostate, called the external urethral sphincter,

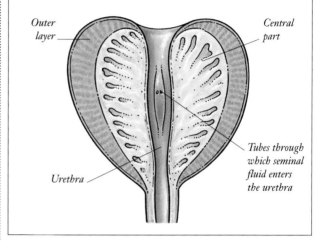

Inside the Prostate Gland

As this diagram shows, the prostate gland consists of a central part and an outer layer. The two parts are affected by different diseases of the prostate.

Outer layer

Central part

Tubes through which seminal fluid enters the urethra

Urethra

is particularly important in preventing the leakage of urine from the bladder.

▬ WHAT CAUSES THE SYMPTOMS? ▬

As a man gets older, his prostate usually becomes larger. Most of this enlargement takes place after the age of 50. The fact that the prostate grows is not important in itself, and the trouble the growth causes does not depend on its actual size. However, the prostate surrounds the tube from the bladder, called the urethra, that conveys urine out of the body. As the prostate enlarges, it squeezes the urethra and narrows the opening out of the bladder. This obstruction results in slowing the flow of urine.

Effects of an Enlarged Prostate

As the prostate increases in size, it begins to squeeze the urethra, the tube through which urine must pass in order for the bladder to empty. This makes it difficult to urinate and empty the bladder completely.

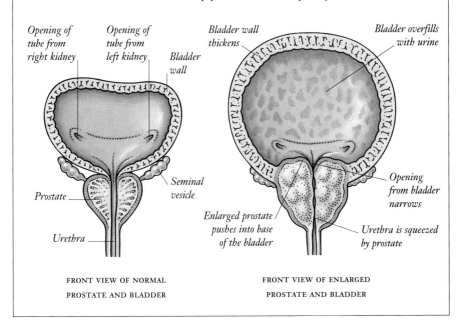

FRONT VIEW OF NORMAL
PROSTATE AND BLADDER

FRONT VIEW OF ENLARGED
PROSTATE AND BLADDER

SYMPTOMS OF OBSTRUCTION

Since obstruction occurs gradually, many men do not realize it is happening. They may notice that their urine stream does not travel as far as it did when they were younger, and they may be aware that it is less forceful. As their condition worsens, there may be a delay in getting started, called hesitancy, and the urine stream may trail off at the end, sometimes causing troublesome dribbling. They may feel that there is still urine in the bladder, which is referred to as incomplete emptying.

Obstructive Symptoms

When the enlargement of the prostate directly obstructs the bladder, the following symptoms are likely to occur.

HESITANCY	Having to wait for the urine to start flowing.
POOR STREAM	The urine flows with less force and projects only a short distance outward.
TERMINAL DRIBBLING	The flow of urine continues after the main stream has finished, sometimes in spurts or dribbles. Occasionally, a second large volume of urine is passed, sometimes called double voiding.
INCOMPLETE EMPTYING	The feeling that there is still urine in the bladder after urination has finished.

HOW IRRITATIVE SYMPTOMS DEVELOP

The obstructive symptoms described above may not be too troublesome. However, the bladder has to work harder to overcome the obstruction and may cause irritative symptoms. Men who are affected by the problem need to urinate more often (frequency), with a feeling of urgency that can become so bad that wetting occurs. If these symptoms occur during the night (nocturia), loss of sleep can become a problem.

This can be a great nuisance to a man who may have to avoid long trips or plan activities around ready access to toilet facilities. The problem may also affect family, friends, and colleagues, who may not be sympathetic. In fact, friends and relatives may be more aware of the problem than the sufferer, who unconsciously adjusts his activities and lifestyle and accepts the symptoms as inevitable. Often, a patient is sent to seek treatment by his wife, whose sleep is interrupted by his constant trips to the bathroom.

ACUTE RETENTION OF URINE

Sometimes a man with an enlarged prostate will quite suddenly be unable to urinate. The bladder fills up and becomes very painful. This is called acute retention.

Irritative Symptoms

The effect on the bladder of having to work harder to overcome obstruction can produce the following symptoms.

FREQUENCY	An abnormally short time between urinating.
NOCTURIA	Being awakened in the night by the need to urinate.
URGENCY	Being unable to hold on after feeling the need to urinate. Can lead to leaking of urine, or incontinence.
INCOMPLETE EMPTYING	With irritative symptoms, a sensation of incomplete bladder emptying sometimes occurs, even though the bladder is empty.

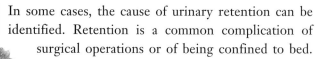

In some cases, the cause of urinary retention can be identified. Retention is a common complication of surgical operations or of being confined to bed. Retention can also be caused by constipation.

Some men develop retention if their bladders become too full. This might occur, for example, on a long trip. Hospitals located on highways that are plagued with traffic jams sometimes admit men with retention. This problem can be prevented by using long-distance buses that have toilets and taking regular rest breaks on long trips.

Cold weather is another problem. Urinary retention sometimes occurs in men attending sports events, when, perhaps after a few beers, there is a long line at the men's room. Large drinks, especially alcoholic ones, may fill the bladder unusually quickly. Drugs called diuretics, which are prescribed to remove excess fluid from the body in heart or chest conditions, also sometimes cause retention. More commonly, medications used to treat the symptoms of the common cold or flu, such as antihistamines, can trigger acute urinary retention.

However, retention often occurs for no apparent reason, and it may occur in men who have previously had only minor obstructive symptoms. Why this happens is not really understood.

PARTNER PRESSURE
You may not notice that you are getting up more often in the night to urinate, but your partner may well find her sleep being disturbed.

CHRONIC RETENTION OF URINE

Painless or chronic retention of urine occurs over months or years as the bladder slowly expands until it may reach four or five times its normal size. Men are not usually aware that this is happening, but sometimes the overfilled bladder leaks urine, causing wetness. In rare cases, the pressure in the bladder grows and damages the kidneys.

Although most men with prostate disorders are unlikely to develop kidney failure, proper treatment in the early stages will usually clear up possible kidney problems completely. It is important that tests be done to rule out the bladder as the source of kidney dysfunction.

OTHER COMPLICATIONS

If the bladder cannot empty completely, urine that remains may become infected or form crystals that grow into bladder stones. The infection may cause a burning sensation, called dysuria, when urine is passed.

Repeated infections may require a prostate operation, but sometimes they are a symptom of prostatitis (see pp.75–77).

Sometimes a large prostate gland bleeds. However, bleeding is more likely to be caused by something other than enlargement and must always be investigated. Very occasionally, repeated bleeding is a reason for operating on the prostate.

— WHY THE PROSTATE ENLARGES —

Most prostate enlargement is due to harmless growth of the prostate tissue and is part of the normal aging process. Enlargement may also be caused by prostatic cancer or an inflammation of the prostate.

BENIGN PROSTATIC HYPERPLASIA

In the majority of men, a condition called benign prostatic hyperplasia, or BPH, causes the prostate to become enlarged. This noncancerous enlargement occurs with aging, and the changes are visible under a microscope.

The exact cause of such enlargement is uncertain. However, the growth requires male hormones and does not occur in men who are sterilized at an early age. Most men over 80 years old have the condition, and about half will have some related symptoms.

As the prostate gland enlarges, both the epithelium and the stroma grow (see pp.10–11). Sometimes the overall size of the gland does not increase very much, and symptoms appear to be caused by the muscle contractions in the stroma that constrict the bladder opening and urethra.

BPH starts in the inner part of the gland (see p.11). The growth compresses the outer part of the gland into a fairly thin shell, which is then called a capsule. BPH never spreads outside the gland. Whatever the dimensions of the growth, the prostate remains covered by the capsule, like a chestnut in its shell. When a doctor examines a prostate gland affected by BPH, it has a smooth surface with an even shape and feels rubbery rather than hard. Unless BPH causes the sort of symptoms described earlier in this chapter, the patient himself does not notice anything unusual. Simply having a large prostate may not produce symptoms, and the prostate gland seems to function normally.

PROSTATITIS

Prostatitis, inflammation of the prostate from infection or other causes, is not uncommon and can occur at almost any age. Sometimes prostatitis causes symptoms such as dysuria, burning pain while urinating. In older men who are already suffering from BPH, prostatitis may cause a sudden increase in prostatic symptoms.

Prostatitis may cause vague symptoms and be difficult to diagnose. There is more information about prostatitis later in the book (see pp.75–77).

Prostatic Cancer

Cancer of the prostate most commonly affects the outer layer of the gland, but as a tumor grows and spreads to the central part, it will obstruct the urethra.

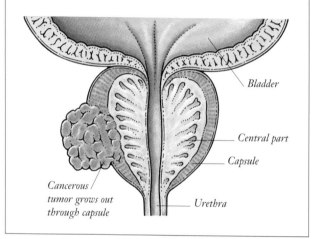

Bladder

Central part

Capsule

Cancerous tumor grows out through capsule

Urethra

CANCER OF THE PROSTATE

The prostate is one of the organs that can develop cancerous tumors. These usually develop in the outer part of the gland (see p.11) and may not block the urethra at first. Surrounding this outer part of the gland is a thin layer of tissue. This layer is also known as a capsule, although it is not the capsule caused by BPH. Many men with tumors also coincidently have BPH in the inner part of the gland. Evaluation of symptoms of BPH often leads to discovery of cancer.

At first the tumor remains inside the outer capsule of the prostate. However, as the tumor enlarges, it spreads through the capsule and grows into the tissue around the prostate. The tumor may also spread if cells break

Microscopic Image of Cancerous Prostate Tissue

In this microscope image of a tissue sample from a prostate tumor magnified over 400 times, a mass of rapidly dividing cancerous cells can be identified by the dark nuclei of the cells, which have absorbed a purple stain applied to the tissue.

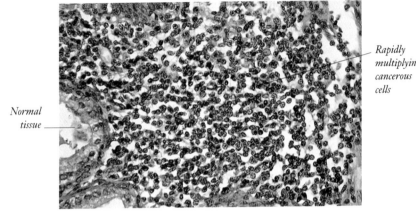

Rapidly multiplying cancerous cells

Normal tissue

away from it. These cells are trapped by the lymph glands near the prostate and may grow into secondary tumors, which are known as metastases. The tumor can also spread along the blood vessels, usually to the bones of the back and pelvis.

A doctor will suspect a tumor if there is a hard lump in the prostate or if the whole prostate feels hard and the shape is uneven. Very small tumors, however, may be impossible to feel.

KEY POINTS

- Symptoms due to prostate problems may be either obstructive or irritative.
- The main disorders of the prostate gland are benign prostatic hyperplasia (BPH), prostatitis, and prostate cancer.

Other conditions causing "prostate symptoms"

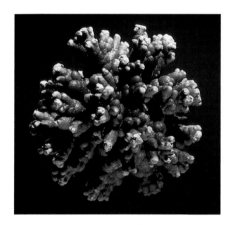

BLADDER STONE
A large stone, seen here magnified, can cause obstruction of the urinary tract, making urination difficult and producing symptoms similar to those of a prostate disorder.

Although we talk about "prostate symptoms," trouble with urination can be due to all sorts of things. Doctors need to do special tests to confirm that the prostate is causing the trouble before they recommend a treatment.

OBSTRUCTION

Men suffering from urethral stricture, bladder stones, or bladder tumors may experience symptoms similar to those of prostate problems.

URETHRAL STRICTURE

Apart from benign prostatic hyperplasia (BPH), the condition most likely to cause blockage is a urethral stricture, a narrowed scarred area that can occur anywhere from just below the prostate to just inside the penis.

Strictures can result from injury, either from a direct blow or from a fracture of the pelvis, or by infection, including sexually transmitted disease. They can also be

Side View of a Urethral Stricture

A stricture of the urethra, caused by scar tissue thickening the wall of the urethra and narrowing the passageway for urine, can result from a physical injury.

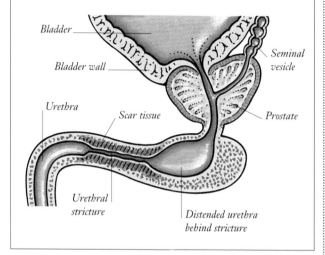

Bladder

Bladder wall

Urethra

Scar tissue

Seminal vesicle

Prostate

Urethral stricture

Distended urethra behind stricture

caused by the placement of a small tube or catheter in the bladder, often done after major surgery, or may develop after prostate surgery.

The event leading to stricture might have occurred many years before. Think about this before your appointment with your doctor or surgeon in case you are asked. Strictures can occur at any age and are suspected more strongly when someone has prostatic symptoms at a younger age than is usual.

BLADDER STONES AND TUMORS

A stone in the bladder might cause a sudden blockage, either producing retention of urine or intermittently severe symptoms. However, a bladder stone can also be a complication of BPH because a constantly filled bladder that does not empty completely leads to the formation of bladder stones.

Very rarely, a tumor in the bladder may grow down into the prostate and cause it to enlarge, but this is usually associated with other symptoms such as bleeding.

═══ NONOBSTRUCTIVE SYMPTOMS ═══

Prostate symptoms should not simply be dismissed as due to "old age" because they could be due to other causes. As people get older, all of their bodily functions, including emptying the bladder, can deteriorate. Irritative symptoms, such as frequency or urgency, can occur without obstruction.

One common problem is the need to urinate during the night, which affects elderly women as much as elderly men. Many men who have prostate operations are disappointed to find that afterward they still have to get up in the night. Older people tend to sleep less well; they urinate because they are awake or sleeping less deeply, rather than being awakened by the need to urinate. Sometimes the kidneys are not as good at restricting the amount of urine made in the night. Some drugs also increase the amount of urine.

Some diseases, such as diabetes, can develop in old age, increasing urine production and affecting the number of times the bladder needs to be emptied. Some diseases of the nervous system, including strokes and Parkinson's disease, can also affect the bladder.

A change in lifestyle may also cause trouble. After they retire from employment, many men drink more tea, coffee, or alcohol than they did while working.

More fluid in means more fluid out. Therefore, a man needs to urinate more often.

Trouble with the bladder is not an inevitable consequence of getting old. However, even when bladder trouble stems from the prostate, a prostate operation is not an infallible cure for every urinary symptom. Surgery can actually make things worse in some cases. Before undergoing treatment, a patient should have his condition thoroughly assessed. The next chapter explains what procedures are used to do this, why they are done, and what the results mean.

BLOOD IN THE URINE

Blood in the urine (hematuria) should not be considered a "prostate symptom." As many as one-third of the men with this symptom who are seen by urologists have something potentially serious, such as a tumor in the bladder or the kidney.

Many of these tumors are not cancerous and can be cured. In all cases, the sooner a tumor is diagnosed, the more likely it is to be cured and the easier treatment is likely to be.

Blood in the urine is investigated using cystoscopy (see pp.35–36) and either an X-ray procedure called an intravenous urogram or an ultrasound scan (see pp.32–33). If you see blood in your urine, do not ignore it even if it goes away. You should see your primary care physician or urologist immediately.

Sometimes, blood that is not visible to the naked eye is detected when a urine specimen is tested. Although this is less likely than visible bleeding to be caused by something serious, it is still best to have it investigated by your physician or urologist.

KEY POINTS

- Urethral strictures, bladder stones, and bladder tumors can all cause "prostate symptoms."
- Symptoms can also be caused by deteriorating bodily functions associated with old age and changes in lifestyle.

Investigating the prostate

If you are a man at the right age for prostate problems and have read this far, you are probably wondering whether you need to have your prostate examined.

Answer the questions in the table on page 29 and add up your score. A low score will indicate that you have mild symptoms of benign prostate hyperplasia, while a high score will show that you have severe symptoms for which you should receive treatment.

First, consult your primary care physician. If you appear to have a prostate problem, you will usually be referred to a urologist, a surgeon who specializes in diseases of the kidneys, the bladder, and the male sexual organs, as well as the prostate. The urologist will determine whether your symptoms are caused by enlargement of the prostate, if the enlargement is benign, and

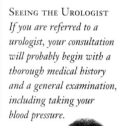

SEEING THE UROLOGIST
If you are referred to a urologist, your consultation will probably begin with a thorough medical history and a general examination, including taking your blood pressure.

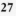

what treatment, if any, is needed. The doctor will ask you various questions, give you a physical examination, and arrange for special tests.

SEEING A DOCTOR

A doctor needs to know as much as possible about a patient's symptoms to make the correct diagnosis and decide if and how the condition should be treated. Think about your symptoms carefully before you see the doctor, since it will help you answer questions.

It is also important to tell the doctor why you are concerned about your symptoms. Some men simply want to be reassured that their symptoms are not a sign of something serious. If all seems well, they may not want to be treated. Other men have such uncomfortable symptoms that they are desperate to have them treated.

If you are simply worried and want reassurance, do not be afraid to say so. Your honesty will avoid a misunderstanding that could lead to the wrong advice.

SYMPTOM QUESTIONNAIRES

Your doctor may use a set of standard questions from a printed list or may use a computer. In some hospitals, you may be given the questionnaire beforehand. If so, someone will go through the questions and discuss with you anything that is not clear. The questions are designed to find out the problem and the severity of the symptoms. The severity is assigned a number, and the numbers for all the questions can then be added up to give a "score" that measures the seriousness of the problem. Questions about your general health are also important, especially if an operation is being considered.

Prostate Self-Assessment Questions

A questionnaire has been devised to help both you and your doctor to determine the severity of your prostate symptoms. Answer each of the questions and add up your score. A score of 0–8 indicates mild symptoms of benign prostate hyperplasia; 9–19, moderate symptoms; and 20–35, severe symptoms.

	NOT AT ALL	LESS THAN 1 TIME IN 5	LESS THAN HALF THE TIME	HALF THE TIME	MORE THAN HALF THE TIME	ALMOST ALWAYS
Over the past month, how often have you had a sensation of not emptying your bladder completely after you finished urinating?	0	1	2	3	4	5
Over the past month, how often have you had to urinate again less than 2 hours after you last urinated?	0	1	2	3	4	5
Over the past month, on how many occasions have you started and stopped urinating several times before you were done?	0	1	2	3	4	5
Over the past month, how often have you found it difficult to postpone urination?	0	1	2	3	4	5
Over the past month, how often have you had a weak urinary stream?	0	1	2	3	4	5
Over the past month, how often have you had to push or strain to begin urination?	0	1	2	3	4	5
	NONE	1 TIME	2 TIMES	3 TIMES	4 TIMES	5 TIMES OR MORE
Over the past month, how many times did you most typically get up to urinate from the time you went to bed at night until the time you got up in the morning?	0	1	2	3	4	5

Courtesy of the American Urological Association

HAVING AN EXAMINATION

You will need to have both a general examination and a prostate examination. Your abdomen will be checked to make sure that your bladder is not enlarged. Your penis and testes will be examined. Sometimes narrowing of the opening in the foreskin, known as phimosis, can cause symptoms similar to those arising from conditions of the prostate. A circumcision may be all that is needed.

The final part of the examination is feeling the prostate gland itself. The doctor can do this only by putting his finger into your rectum (the digital rectal exam). Many men are worried and anxious about the exam, and this is why they sometimes do not admit to having prostate symptoms.

Apprehension about this type of examination is natural. The doctor realizes that it is embarrassing and will do it as discreetly as possible. You should tell the doctor if you have a problem affecting your anus, such as hemorrhoids or pain when you defecate.

Usually, you will be asked to lie on your left side, although some doctors prefer another position. Relax as much as possible. Bending your knees makes it easier for the doctor to feel your prostate. The doctor wears a thin soft glove on which he puts some jelly to allow the finger to enter the rectum easily.

The examination usually takes only a few seconds and allows the doctor to determine the size of your prostate and sometimes suggests the cause if there is enlargement. Normally, the prostate is not tender. If prostatitis is suspected, you may be asked whether touching the prostate is painful. In some cases, the prostate may be massaged during the examination so that fluid can be passed through the urethra for analysis. The rectum itself may also be examined.

UNDERGOING TESTS

Knowing your symptoms and their severity, as well as the condition of your prostate and your overall health, the doctor will usually have a sense of the problem but will want to perform tests to confirm this and to plan treatment. Some tests are done in nearly all cases, others only in certain situations.

You will be asked for a sample of your urine. This may be collected when the flow test is done (see below). A blood sample is usually taken to check how your kidneys are working and to measure a substance called prostate-specific antigen (PSA). The blood test results are usually available in a few days.

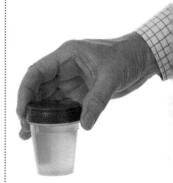

PROVIDING A SAMPLE
After your examination, the doctor will usually ask you to provide a urine sample for laboratory analysis.

URINE FLOW MEASUREMENT

When the prostate is obstructing the bladder opening, it will slow down the passage of urine. Machines that measure urine flow are used to test for obstruction. The test is very simple. You urinate into a funnel-shaped container just as if you were using a toilet. All the measurements are done automatically.

However, the test is only accurate if a fairly large amount of urine is passed. Drink plenty of fluid before going to the hospital so that you arrive with your bladder comfortably full. If you are not able to do this, you will be given water to drink and asked to wait until your bladder has filled before the test is performed. If you are in the waiting room and need to urinate, tell one of the staff. You may be able to do the flow test right away.

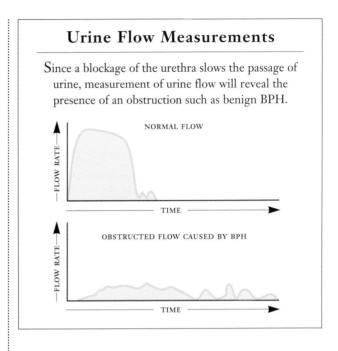

Urine Flow Measurements

Since a blockage of the urethra slows the passage of urine, measurement of urine flow will reveal the presence of an obstruction such as benign BPH.

NORMAL FLOW

FLOW RATE

TIME

OBSTRUCTED FLOW CAUSED BY BPH

FLOW RATE

TIME

Sometimes, when first doing the test, you may pass only a little urine. If this happens and you later feel the urge to urinate again, do not go to the toilet. Tell one of the staff and use the flow machine again. When you are urinating into the machine, try to relax. Straining will affect the reading. Try to keep the urine stream in one direction. Letting it "wander around" may result in a false reading. Also, you should avoid bumping against the machine during use. These precautions will help produce an accurate record to determine whether obstruction is present.

X-RAYS AND ULTRASOUND

Men with prostate disease used to have an X-ray called an intravenous urogram (IVU), which involved the injection of a dye that allowed the kidneys to show up on the X-ray. Now, an IVU is done only in certain circumstances, such as when blood is seen in the urine.

A simple X-ray of your abdomen can be useful and is particularly good at detecting a stone in either the bladder or the kidneys. It also may show the size of the bladder. Therefore, the X-ray is usually done after urinating, perhaps immediately after the flow test, to check how completely the bladder empties.

An ultrasound scan provides an easy way to look at the kidneys. A doctor or technician simply runs a small transducer over the back and front of your abdomen. Ultrasound can also be used to measure how well your bladder is emptying. This examination is called a postvoid residual urine determination and can be done at the same time as your kidney scan. However, there are also small portable machines designed just for this purpose that might be used by either the doctor or nurse.

■ UNDERGOING ADDITIONAL TESTS ■

The tests described above are performed on most men with prostate trouble. In certain circumstances, other tests are needed. As mentioned above, an intravenous urogram may be used if bleeding has occurred, kidney stones are suspected, or an abnormality in the kidney is found on an ultrasound scan (see p.25).

TRANSRECTAL ULTRASOUND SCAN

A transrectal ultrasound scan employs a metal probe that is gently passed into the rectum, allowing examination of the inside of the prostate. If necessary, a fine needle can be passed through the probe and into the prostate to take small pieces of tissue for microscopic examination in a process called needle biopsy. Transrectal ultrasound scanning is done either if an accurate measurement of the size of the prostate is needed or if prostate cancer is suspected. Some urology clinics have a portable machine for this test and use it on most patients with prostate disorders.

CYSTOMETROGRAM

Sometimes a test called a cystometrogram, or urodynamics, is needed. A small tube called a catheter is passed through the urethra to measure the pressure inside the bladder, which is filled with fluid.

In some cases, this test shows spasms of increased pressure, a condition called an "unstable bladder," which is one of the causes of frequency and urgency. This condition can develop when BPH obstructs the urethra. There is a good chance of improvement after an operation on the prostate. There are other reasons, however, for an unstable bladder. If the problem is not caused by BPH, a prostate operation will not cure it and might even make the symptoms worse.

Measuring the pressure during urination is also important. Poor flow (see p.32) is usually caused by obstruction due to BPH. In this case, the bladder has to work very hard to produce a pressure high enough to maintain an adequate flow rate. Then a prostate operation may be necessary. However, sometimes a poor flow of urine results not because of obstruction by the prostate but because the bladder itself is weak. In this case, the bladder pressure will be less than normal. This condition will not be improved by an operation on the prostate.

Having a cystometrogram may be unpleasant. The procedure involves having a catheter passed into your bladder and another tube into the rectum, both of which are attached to a recording machine. It may be uncomfortable to have the bladder filled and then urinate with the tube still in the bladder. For this reason, the procedure is usually performed only when a prostate operation is being considered or when results from the other simpler tests are not completely clear. However, the test results help prevent the use of inappropriate treatments.

A newer method of performing a cystometrogram is available, in which the tubes are connected to a small portable device attached to a belt. The patient can remain mobile, and measurements are recorded for several hours as the bladder fills and empties naturally during normal activities. This is called ambulatory urodynamics and may be used more in the future.

CYSTOSCOPY

Examining the bladder and prostate with a camera-like instrument called a cystoscope may also be important in some circumstances. A cystoscopy is essential if there has been blood in the urine. It may be advised if symptoms are mainly irritative and might be due to some condition in the bladder itself. The urethra is also examined to rule out a urethral stricture.

Some surgeons find cystoscopy helpful in planning an operation. In the past, when only rigid metal cystoscopes were available, general anesthesia was usually given. Now, the urologist often uses a flexible cystoscope that can be passed into the bladder through the urethra with very little discomfort. A jelly containing local anesthetic is used to numb the urethra.

The examination takes a few minutes, and, if video equipment is available, the patient can see inside his own bladder during the test. To improve the view, fluid is poured into the bladder through a tube in the cystoscope during the examination. This may feel a little cold, and the bladder will feel full. Do not worry about having an accident. You probably will not, but, even if you do, the examination area is designed to accommodate such accidents. You will be asked to urinate after the test is completed. If you cannot urinate, or if you feel that you have not emptied your bladder properly, tell the medical staff. Do not go home until you are comfortable.

After a cystometrogram or cystoscopy you may be sore, feel burning after urination, or see some blood in your urine. This goes away quickly, especially if you drink plenty of fluid for a few days. If these symptoms persist or if you have difficulty urinating, call the urologist or see your doctor.

KEY POINTS

- A prostate operation is not a cure for every urinary symptom. Before treatment, the condition must be thoroughly assessed.
- The doctor will ask questions and perform a physical examination and tests to determine the cause of your symptoms.
- Some of the tests, such as cystoscopy, may cause discomfort and some blood in the urine for a day or two.

How is BPH treated?

Until recently, the only palliative treatment for benign prostatic hyperplasia was an operation. If your symptoms are not too bad, you probably just need reassurance that the condition is not dangerous. You also need simple advice about the amount of fluid to drink, the time needed to empty the bladder, and learning to live with minor symptoms.

Why is treatment not always given? One answer is that there is always a risk of side effects from any treatment, whether surgery or drugs. If the symptoms are mild, the side effects could be worse than the condition itself. Research has shown that prostate operations are usually very successful if the patient has been suffering from severe symptoms, but many men who have only mild symptoms are disappointed with the results.

Surgery remains the most effective method of treating

SIMPLE MEASURES
Taking such steps as drinking enough liquid or not drinking too much can help improve the symptoms of BPH.

37

BPH. An operation, rather than some other type of treatment, is essential if the patient has had retention of urine or if obstruction has caused kidney failure. Sometimes tests indicate severe obstruction. An operation can then prevent a complication such as kidney failure. If the symptoms are very bad, an operation is usually the best way to improve them. Even if the symptoms are milder, surgery may be the only appropriate treatment if tests have shown that the prostate is causing severe obstruction.

Compared with some types of surgery, prostate operations are very safe. Men with serious health problems can have a prostate operation without danger. However, an operation is not advisable in someone who is older or very out of shape unless he is experiencing a lot of problems.

Whether an operation is necessary often depends on how badly the symptoms affect the patient. Unless BPH causes a risk to your health, which is unusual, the urologist may discuss the possibility of surgery with you but leave the final decision up to you.

TYPES OF SURGERY

The earliest operations on the prostate were done as "open" surgery, in which the enlarged part of the gland was removed through a surgical incision. Today, if the gland is very large, this operation is still the best method and is usually very successful.

However, just before World War II, urologists in the US started using a procedure called transurethral resection of the prostate, or TURP. It was one of the earliest types of operations using minimally invasive, or "keyhole" surgery. Now nearly all prostate operations

Performing a Transurethral Resection

A resectoscope, which is inserted through the urethra, enables the surgeon to see the enlarged prostate and then cut away and remove the part of the gland that is causing the obstruction.

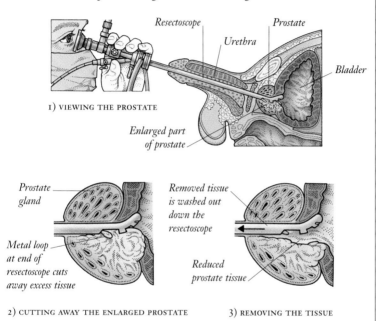

Resectoscope

Prostate

Urethra

Bladder

1) VIEWING THE PROSTATE

Enlarged part of prostate

Prostate gland

Removed tissue is washed out down the resectoscope

Metal loop at end of resectoscope cuts away excess tissue

Reduced prostate tissue

2) CUTTING AWAY THE ENLARGED PROSTATE   3) REMOVING THE TISSUE

are done this way. An instrument called a resectoscope is passed into the prostate through the urethra. The urologist can see the prostate through the scope and uses a special type of electrified metal loop to remove part or all of the prostate in pieces. Once the enlarged prostate has been cut away, any bleeding blood vessels are sealed with an electric current. The result is a cavity in the middle of the gland through which urine will pass easily.

Although the sphincter muscle around the neck of the bladder is cut away (opposite), the surgeon will take great care not to injure the external bladder sphincter below the prostate. The control of the flow of urine after a TURP procedure is usually good. The raw cavity left after the operation soon develops a protective lining called epithelium.

The surgery usually takes about half an hour. General anesthesia may be used, but the operation is often done with the patient awake but numb from the waist down from a spinal anesthetic given in the back. Many surgeons now use a small television camera to project a picture of the operation on a screen, and the patient may be able to watch if he chooses.

If you are to have a TURP, you will probably be admitted to the hospital on the day of the surgery. A final physical examination, some blood tests, and other tests, including a chest X-ray, may be carried out several days before the surgery. The urologist and anesthesiologist will discuss the operation with you. You may be given a choice between general and spinal anesthesia. For men with certain conditions, such as pulmonary disease, general anesthesia may not be advisable.

AFTER THE OPERATION

Transurethral resection requires only a brief hospital stay, usually 1–2 days. Since the TURP procedure does not involve a surgical incision, postoperative pain is considerably less than it is in more invasive types of surgery.

BLEEDING

After the operation, a flexible tube called a catheter is put into the bladder to drain the urine and is usually removed

The Results of a Complete Resection

Resection cuts away all of the central part of the prostate gland, removing the enlarged part of the gland, increasing the width of the urethra, and allowing the urine to flow normally.

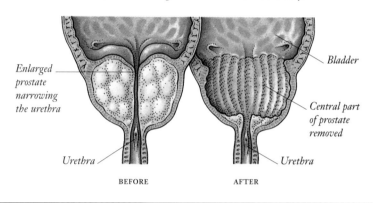

Enlarged prostate narrowing the urethra

Bladder

Central part of prostate removed

Urethra

Urethra

BEFORE   AFTER

within two days. Although the urologist controls most of the bleeding at the end of the operation, some blood does drain with the urine. There can be a lot of blood for a day or two. Occasionally, the blood clots and blocks the catheter. If this happens, a doctor or nurse clears out the catheter with a syringe. Many urologists use special catheters to run fluid through the bladder to reduce the risk of clotting.

WILL IT BE PAINFUL?

You will not have any of the usual type of postoperative pain, but the catheter can be uncomfortable, making the bladder feel full. Occasionally, painful spasms occur. If these are severe, drugs can be prescribed to control them. You will be asked to drink a lot of water each day to help flush out your bladder.

RETURNING TO NORMAL LIFE

Once the catheter is removed, you should be able to urinate again almost at once. It is normal to need to urinate more frequently than usual for a day or two, and often it is difficult to control the flow at first. A therapist or nurse will teach you some exercises to help control urination. Most men go home soon after the catheter is removed. Sometimes it is difficult to urinate initially. Persevering for a few hours usually does the trick. If you cannot urinate, the catheter may need to be reinserted. If this happens, do not worry; everything is usually fine when the catheter is taken out again.

Although there is no painful incision on the body's exterior, the prostate is raw and needs time to heal. The healing takes a few weeks. It is important to take it easy during this time. Continue to drink plenty of fluids but not alcohol. Avoid heavy lifting and do not drive for 2–3 weeks. Sexual intercourse should also be avoided during this period. You can expect to see some bits of tissue in the urine from time to time. This is like the scab coming off a skin wound. As sometimes happens when a scab comes off, a little bleeding may occur.

Traces of blood in the urine are very common after a prostate operation. Occasionally, heavier bleeding occurs, usually 1–2 weeks after the operation. Do not panic if this happens; a little blood goes a long way in the urine and often looks worse than it is. Drink plenty of fluid, and, if the bleeding does not stop in a few hours, contact your doctor.

In some cases blood clots make urination difficult and require a return to the hospital to have a catheter replaced for a day or two. Such bleeding usually resolves itself, or if due to an infection, antibiotics are given.

Since BPH develops slowly in most men over some years, a man may be surprised by the force of his urine stream after a TURP. Usually, this is immediately obvious. However, when frequency is the main symptom, the condition may take longer to improve and may not return completely to normal. Needing to urinate at night may persist after the operation because this symptom is often as much a feature of aging as of actual prostate disease. The other symptom that may not improve is leakage at the end of urinating. Indeed, some men notice this for the first time after the operation. Urine leaks out from the cavity inside the prostate. It can usually be controlled by taking a little care when urinating.

Something that almost always happens after the operation is what doctors call "retrograde ejaculation." At the end of sexual intercourse, a normal climax is felt, but nothing comes out. During the operation, the muscle at the neck of the bladder, above the prostate, is removed with the prostate tissue. As a result, semen leaks into the bladder rather than coming out normally. Usually, sex is otherwise unaffected. However, a few men experience difficulty in having an erection after the operation.

After a prostate operation, your control of urine should be normal, although, if your preoperative symptoms were of the irritative type, leakage may occur at first. You may need medication to calm your bladder, often only as a temporary measure. More rarely, the lower sphincter muscle is weakened by the surgery. This usually improves with muscle strengthening exercises and is rarely permanent. Corrective surgery can be done if all else fails. Leakage occasionally occurs if an insufficient amount of prostate has been removed and the bladder does not empty completely. If so, a second TURP might be needed.

Men who have had a TURP are among the most satisfied patients seen in a urology office. The majority are delighted with the operation. The few who are disappointed with the results are usually those whose symptoms were fairly mild before the operation and who find that the side effects are worse than their original symptoms.

A poor result of a TURP usually indicates that the operation was not the best treatment for the patient rather than anything having gone wrong with the operation. As previously stated, you should have the right tests done beforehand and decide if your symptoms are worth the discomfort of an operation and the risk of side effects. Above all, go to a urologist with the expectation of receiving helpful advice but not necessarily having an operation.

DRUG TREATMENTS

For men with prostate symptoms who are not severely affected, do not want to consider surgery, or are not well enough for an operation, there is an alternative. BPH can now by treated with drugs. There are two types of drugs: one makes the prostate smaller, and the other relaxes the muscle in the prostate and bladder neck. Both drugs can reduce the obstruction caused by the prostate sufficiently to relieve symptoms.

HORMONES

The drugs that shrink the prostate interfere with the action of the male hormone testosterone, which is part of the cause of BPH. This interference reverses the condition, and the prostate shrinks. Since male hormones work in a different way in other organs, this type of drug affects only the prostate and is almost completely free of side effects.

A number of these drugs are being developed, but only one, finasteride, is available now. It is given as a single pill once a day. It may take three months or more for the prostate to shrink enough to improve symptoms. Finasteride is prescribed as a long-term treatment. Do not stop taking it after a week or two even if symptoms do not seem to be improving. Finasteride is very safe and free from major side effects, although a small number of men experience erectile dysfunction or other sexual difficulties. This usually improves if the drug is stopped. If sexual intercourse is very important to you, this treatment may not be the right one. However, sexual problems are more common following a TURP and are not reversible in that case. The other important point about finasteride is that, as soon as the drug is stopped, the prostate grows again very rapidly. Once this drug works, you need to keep taking it.

ALPHA-BLOCKER DRUGS

The other type of drug used to treat BPH is called an alpha-blocker. Contraction of muscle in the prostate narrows the bladder opening and increases obstruction caused by BPH. Alpha-blockers improve symptoms by relaxing the muscle and reducing the obstruction. These drugs, unfortunately, affect muscle and blood vessels in other parts of the body and can cause side effects such as faintness, weakness, and lethargy.

Alpha-blockers are also used to treat high blood pressure, but some of the newer ones seem to act more on the prostate than on other organs and may have fewer side effects. Their big advantage is that they work almost immediately. Doxazosin, prazosin, tamsulosin, and terazosin are now in use, and other alpha-blockers will be introduced soon. They differ in how often they are taken, and some need to be increased gradually from a low dose. Their side effects also differ. If one is not suitable, it is worth trying another. Alpha-blockers can cause retrograde ejaculation, but this reverts to normal if the drug is stopped. As with hormone treatment, alpha-blockers only slightly improve the rate of urinary flow.

CHOICE OF DRUG

The choice of finasteride or alpha-blockers depends on a number of things. Some men, often those whose symptoms occur at a fairly young age, do not have much actual enlargement of the prostate. For them, the action of the prostatic muscle seems to be the main cause of the obstruction, and an alpha-blocker is therefore the best choice.

If a man with a relatively normal-size prostate gland does need an operation, the surgeon may not have to cut away any prostate tissue but may just make an incision in one or two places to open it up. The procedure is called transurethral incision of the prostate, or TUIP. The patient will not really be able to tell much difference between having a TUIP and a TURP. This procedure can be performed on men who have a normal-size prostate gland if they do not respond to drug therapy.

Finasteride probably should be prescribed only when the prostate is definitely enlarged. It seems that the bigger the prostate, the more effective finasteride is. Since time is needed to shrink the prostate, the patient must be prepared to wait for the drug to take effect.

To date, the results of combining finasteride with alpha-blocker drugs have been controversial and inconclusive. The National Institutes of Health have conducted trials to compare the effectiveness of combining the drugs to using either of them alone.

Drug treatment is usually suggested if symptoms are mild, the obstruction is not too severe, and there is no reason to avoid using a particular drug. Drugs may be tried in more severe cases if there are medical reasons to avoid surgery. If an operation must be delayed, drugs can be used for temporary help. Some men close to retirement might want to wait until they stop work to have an operation. Teachers, politicians, or other men with fixed vacations might prefer an operation during the summer and find temporary drug treatment helpful. Occasionally, the urologist might suggest trying some drug treatment first to see if it relieves a particular symptom before taking the irreversible step of surgery.

Although these drugs have relieved symptoms in men for whom an operation was not appropriate, there are still many men who are best advised against drug treatment. Drugs should be used only after the prostate has been thoroughly assessed and the tests described earlier (see pp.31–36) have been done. Often this still means seeing a urologist. However, partly as a result of the introduction of drugs to treat BPH, many primary care physicians are becoming more involved in treating the prostate and may prescribe therapy.

OTHER TREATMENTS

Recently, much publicity has been given to heat and laser treatment for BPH. Heat treatment, called "hyperthermia" or "thermotherapy," warms up the prostate. The treatment is given through a probe placed in either the anus or the urethra. Early forms of this treatment warmed the prostate a little and had only a minor effect, although patients' symptoms often improved. It is now possible to heat the prostate a lot more without affecting the surrounding organs, and the results are more promising. The effects are probably closer to those produced by drugs than by a TURP. However, heat treatment is unlikely to become an alternative to TURP for men with severe BPH.

Laser treatment is more like a TURP. It is an alternative way of either removing the enlarged part of the prostate or of cutting it open to widen the outlet. There are a number of different ways of applying laser treatment. Although laser treatment in medicine has received much publicity, urologists have yet to agree on the best way to use lasers on the prostate or even whether laser treatment will prove to be useful in the long run. There is now a similar treatment called vaporization, which involves a slight modification of the resectoscope instrument used in a TURP.

The advantage of many of these treatments is that they can be performed on outpatients, which means that the patient can go home the day the surgery is performed and does not need to spend a night in the hospital. However, the patient often needs to have a catheter in the bladder for several days after treatment. The long-term effects are also uncertain. New is not necessarily better. Although the advantages and disadvantages of these treatments are becoming clearer, most urologists still feel that more testing is needed before they can be generally recommended. This is one reason why such treatments are not widely available.

Another reason is that the equipment is often expensive, and medical facilities want to know how well a treatment works before buying equipment for it. Where such treatments are available, they may be for use in clinical testing or "on trial." Clinical trials for prostate disease are explained further on page 79.

Another form of treatment consists of stents, which are short tubes, usually made of inert metal mesh, that are placed in the prostate to keep it open. A stent can be put in with very little disturbance, often under local anesthesia. A stent might be used to avoid permanent catheterization in a man who is not healthy enough to undergo an operation. However, stents can often cause long-term problems and are rarely used in the US.

KEY POINTS

- Surgery is the most effective way to treat BPH. Transurethral resection of the prostate (TURP) is the operation of choice.
- The benefits of surgery have to be weighed against the side effects and possible complications.
- Drug therapy is available for men whose symptoms are mild, who do not want surgery, or who are not healthy enough for an operation.
- The two main types of drug are those that shrink the prostate (hormones) and those that relax the muscle within the prostate (alpha-blockers).

Urinary retention

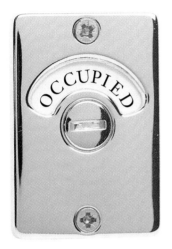

UNCOMFORTABLE DELAY
A man with an enlarged prostate may find that he cannot urinate all at once.

Urinary retention is one of the most unpleasant things that can happen to a man with prostate trouble. He feels the need to urinate, but can force out only a dribble or nothing at all.

As the bladder of a man with prostate problems fills, more and more pain may occur. Occasionally, after a long period of discomfort, something finally flows out, and the condition rights itself. Often, however, it does not. This requires a trip to the hospital to have a catheter put into the bladder to drain the urine. Although this sounds unpleasant, catheterization is effective in relieving symptoms.

CATHETERIZATION

Before a catheter is inserted, jelly containing a local anesthetic is put into the urethra. The jelly numbs the urethra and lubricates it so that catheter insertion is easier. After a short delay to let the anesthetic take effect, the doctor inserts the catheter. There is usually an awkward moment as the catheter goes through the prostate into the bladder, but then relief is instant.

Sometimes the catheter cannot pass through, and a suprapubic catheter is used instead. This type of catheter is put into the bladder through the skin of the lower abdomen under local anesthesia. Since the full bladder is so close to the surface, the procedure is safe and straightforward.

The patient is usually kept in the hospital, although he can go home with the catheter. The catheter may be taken out after a few days, especially if there was an obvious cause of retention, such as constipation, medication, or too much alcohol. Many men can then urinate again. However, retention may indicate that a prostate operation is needed, and, if so, surgery should be done as soon as possible to avoid prolonged catheterization.

How a Catheter Works

Catheterization involves passing a tube up the penis into the bladder and inflating a small balloon to keep it in place. It sounds unpleasant but provides an immediate solution to an uncomfortable condition.

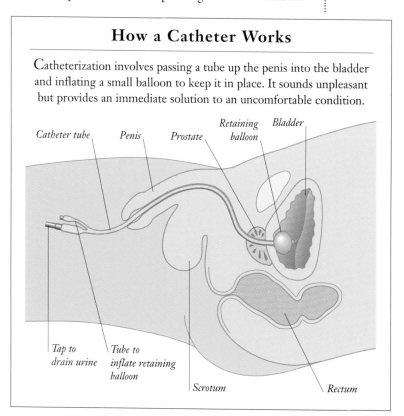

KIDNEY FAILURE

Sometimes, painless chronic retention is associated with with kidney failure. In this case, the treatment is a little little different. A catheter is still necessary, but once the blockage is removed the kidneys start to produce copious amounts of fluid and the catheter must be replaced.

In this case, the administration of intravenous fluid to replace lost volume is usually necessary. Before a prostate operation can be performed, the kidneys must recover, which can take a few weeks.

RESULTS OF TREATMENT

After sudden acute retention, the results of prostate surgery are usually good. In chronic retention, the over-stretched bladder may not work very well and even after an operation may still not empty. Sometimes bladder function improves if a catheter is left in place for a few weeks. Hospitalization is not necessary because it is easy to look after a catheter at home.

KEY POINTS

- Retention of urine can be relieved by insertion of a catheter into the bladder to drain the urine.
- After catheterization for retention, a prostate operation is often necessary.

Prostate-specific antigen

A fairly new blood test, called a prostate-specific antigen (PSA) test, has been given a lot of publicity as a method of early diagnosis of prostate cancer. It is important to understand the test and its implications.

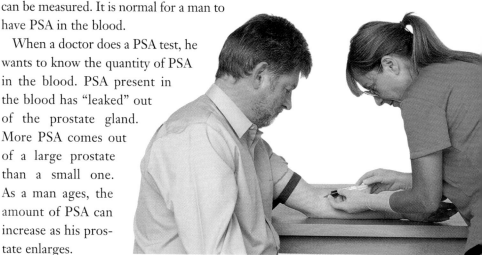

A USEFUL MARKER
A blood test reveals how much PSA the prostate is releasing into the bloodstream, which is a useful indication of activity in the gland.

Prostate-specific antigen is a substance made only by the prostate gland and is part of the fluid that the prostate adds to the semen. Some PSA gets into the blood and can be measured. It is normal for a man to have PSA in the blood.

When a doctor does a PSA test, he wants to know the quantity of PSA in the blood. PSA present in the blood has "leaked" out of the prostate gland. More PSA comes out of a large prostate than a small one. As a man ages, the amount of PSA can increase as his prostate enlarges.

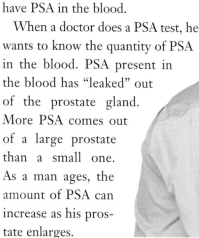

Some diseases of the prostate make the gland more "leaky," and, in this case, the amount of PSA in the blood is even greater. This happens in cancer of the prostate and is the reason the test can be used to look for cancer. Other diseases of the prostate also make it more leaky. For example, a man's PSA level may be high when the prostate is infected. The amount of PSA also goes up after a prostate operation, cystoscopic examination, or catheter insertion.

Since older men have larger prostates and are more prone to noncancerous diseases of the prostate such as prostatitis, the average PSA is higher in men of 75 than in men of 55 years of age. Therefore, if your PSA is higher than normal, it does not necessarily mean that you have cancer. It is more likely that you have BPH or that something else has happened to increase the amount of PSA in your blood.

PSA is helpful as a test for cancer, but the results have to be interpreted carefully. In technical terms, the test is not very specific and gives a lot of false positives, which are results that seem to indicate cancer when it is not

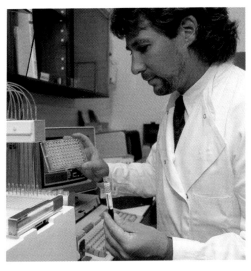

TESTING THE BLOOD
If laboratory analysis of a blood sample shows a very high level of PSA, cancer of the prostate may be suspected.

actually present. If the PSA is very high, however, cancer is likely to be present. If the level is only slightly elevated, the size of the prostate and other conditions affecting the prostate must be taken into account.

Other tests will certainly be necessary before cancer can be diagnosed. The diagnosis of prostate cancer is generally confirmed by a biopsy, the removal of small pieces of prostate tissue with a needle, which is usually done during a transrectal ultrasound scan (see p.33). Sometimes a biopsy of the prostate causes infection in the urine or in the bloodstream. More importantly, the biopsy might miss the tumor; thus, a negative biopsy can sometimes give false assurance. Even if the biopsy is negative, further PSA checks, and even another biopsy, are sometimes necessary. It can be very difficult to be completely certain that an elevated PSA is not caused by cancer.

PSA AND CANCER

In a man who is found to have cancer of the prostate, the amount of PSA is a good indication of the extent of the disease and helps in making treatment decisions. If the PSA is normal or only slightly elevated, it is unlikely that the tumor has spread significantly, which is reassuring. Successful treatment of the cancer lowers the PSA level. However, in all cases, regular determination of the amount of PSA in the blood is an important part of the follow-up. Despite the usefulness of PSA testing, a person with cancer of the prostate can sometimes have a normal PSA test result.

PROSTATE CANCER SCREENING

Cervical smears are used to screen for cancer of the cervix in women. Can PSA be used as a test to screen for cancer of the prostate in the same way in men? This is a difficult question to answer because there is no clear difference between the amount of PSA found in the blood of men with cancer and of men with simple BPH and other benign conditions.

Some men have their PSA level checked once a year. There is no doubt that this detects a lot of cancers that are not causing symptoms. Many of the men who do have cancer have a radical prostatectomy (see p.60), which is becoming one of the most common operations in the US, or undergo radiation therapy or placement of radioactive implants.

Despite the successes of prostate cancer screening, the PSA blood test is not without its gray areas. For every person whose cancer is diagnosed this way, many others have tests done and experience a lot of stress waiting for a negative or inconclusive result. If cancer is found, a radical prostatectomy or radiation therapy will be necessary to treat the cancer. A radical prostatectomy is a serious operation. All of this would be unquestionably worthwhile if it produced a large reduction in the number of men dying from cancer of the prostate. However, some very early cancers grow slowly and in many cases may never cause harm. This is especially the case in older men. It is therefore not clear how many lives are saved. Hence, it may be a good idea to check the PSA in a man over 55 but perhaps less beneficial in men over 75 years of age.

Research into the value of using the PSA test for screening of asymptomatic men is ongoing. If a more specific test were found for prostate cancer, and ways were discovered of deciding which early prostate cancers are dangerous, screening would involve fewer gray areas. The benefits of screening would also be enhanced if there were a simpler method of treatment than radical prostatectomy.

As a general rule, it is wise to measure the PSA level in a man who has prostatic symptoms and/or an abnormality in the prostate on digital rectal examination because these may be due to cancer of the prostate. However, the role of the PSA test in men who have no symptoms or abnormalities on examination is far less clear. It is important that men be fully aware of the possible consequences of an as yet imperfect screening test, especially since the benefits of radical prostatectomy (see pp.63–64) for early cancer remain unclear. A frank and detailed discussion of the pros and cons of PSA screening with your physician is the best way to make the right choice for your particular condition. If prostate cancer is present, different treatment may be required than that used for BPH. The chapter on cancer describes radical prostatectomy for early cancer. Fifteen years ago, this operation was not often done in the US and would have received only a brief mention. The procedure is now part of the regular treatment in urology departments, largely because of earlier diagnosis through PSA testing.

KEY POINTS

- The prostate-specific antigen (PSA) test is a relatively new test for assessing prostate disease.
- Many factors other than cancer can increase the level of PSA in the blood.
- Use of the PSA test is leading to prompt treatment of a greater number of men who have prostate cancer, but the test has limitations.

Prostate cancer

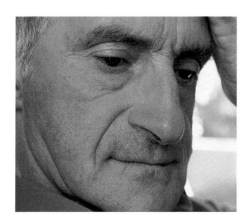

THE OLDER PATIENT
In the elderly, prostate cancer may not alter life expectancy.

Cancer is an alarming word. Many men fear that their prostatic symptoms are caused by cancer. In most cases, this fear is unfounded. However, it is true that cancer of the prostate is quite common.

As with other cancers, prostate cancer can be fatal. However, it is a form of cancer for which several types of treatment are available. In addition, it often grows slowly and may cause little harm, especially in very elderly men.

Recently, doctors have discovered new ways of detecting early cancers in the prostate. Consequently, more men with prostate cancer are being diagnosed at an earlier stage. As mentioned in the last chapter, there is much discussion among cancer specialists about whether these tests should be used for screening in the way that women are screened for breast and cervical cancer (see p.55).

Why cancer of the prostate is so common is not known. In most cases there is no clear family history of prostate cancer, despite the fact that there is a form of the disease that does seem to run in families. If you have only one relative with the disease, do not worry. However, if two or more closely related members of your family have had prostate cancer, particularly if they were young at the time it occurred, you should get your prostate checked every year after you reach age 40 (see p.30). If you have had symptoms suggesting prostate problems, annual checkups should start even earlier. A prostate-specific antigen test should be performed if an abnormality suggesting a possible malignancy is discovered in the course of the digital rectal examination.

Although most authorities agree that screening men without symptoms for prostate cancer with digital rectal examination and/or the prostate-specific antigen test (see pp.53–57) is important, specific recommendations differ among various professional medical organizations and individual physicians. Much of the controversy is centered on the use of the prostate-specific antigen test because the test result can be elevated in noncancerous conditions and subsequent tests to follow up an abnormal reading are invasive and sometimes dangerous.

There are differences in rates of prostate cancer among races and in different parts of the world. Some of this variation may be due to diet or environmental factors. For example, prostate cancer is uncommon in Japan; however, Japanese men who live in the US have a higher risk of developing it. This is probably as a result of differences in diet. Certain types of fatty food may predispose to prostate cancer, whereas other foods, including soy products, may be protective. The data are not yet sufficient to make a determination. However, as doctors understand more about these differences, they may be able to formulate diets that reduce the risk of prostate cancer. Although there was recent concern that vasectomy might make cancer of the prostate more likely, most experts now agree that this is not so.

What Happens in a Radical Prostatectomy?

This operation consists of removing the entire prostate gland and the seminal vesicles and then reconnecting the urethra to the bladder. The procedure is usually performed on younger patients.

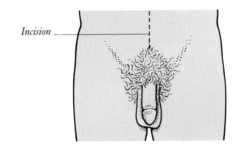

Incision

POINT OF INCISION FOR SURGERY

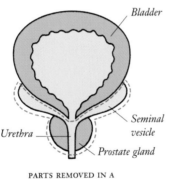

Bladder

Urethra — *Seminal vesicle*

Prostate gland

PARTS REMOVED IN A
RADICAL PROSTATECTOMY

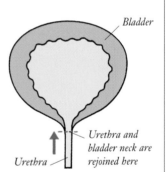

Bladder

Urethra and bladder neck are rejoined here

Urethra

AFTER THE COMPLETION OF A
RADICAL PROSTATECTOMY

═══ HOW IS IT DIAGNOSED? ═══

The difference between cancer of the prostate and benign prostatic hyperplasia (BPH) is that cancer can grow out from the prostate into the surrounding tissues and spread, or metastasize, to other parts of the body, particularly to the bones, causing pain or even fractures.

When cancer is the cause of prostatic symptoms, these complications can recur after treatment if the cancer grows again. Sometimes cancer in the prostate does not cause any prostatic symptoms, and the first sign of the disease can arise in some other part of the body.

Your doctor may suspect that there is a tumor in your prostate if the gland feels abnormally hard or irregular or if your PSA level (see pp.53–57) is particularly high. When any of these symptoms is found, the doctor often arranges for a transrectal ultrasound scan (see p.33). Sometimes, you need an operation called a transurethral resection of the prostate (TURP) because of the severity of your prostate symptoms. Since TURP involves the removal of tissue that can be examined, the procedure is usually done promptly to establish or exclude a diagnosis of cancer. In some cases, cancer is not suspected and is only diagnosed when the tissue removed at an operation is examined by a pathologist.

X-rays or, more typically, a test called a bone scan may be taken to check that there has been no metastasis of the cancer to the bones. This is done by injecting a small amount of a radioactive substance. The substance is absorbed where the bone is active and is detected by a special scanner. A bone scan is not a specific test for cancer, and absorption might be due to other conditions such as arthritis, healed fractures, and benign diseases of the bones. X-rays of the abnormal areas may help. Very occasionally, an orthopedic surgeon might take a small piece of the bone for microscopic examination.

MRI scanning of the pelvis and abdomen is also used to judge the extent of tumor growth and look for disease in regional lymph nodes.

How Is It Treated?

Removing or destroying a cancerous growth cures the disease if the cancer has not spread. Until recently, removal was the only treatment for most cancers. If metastases had already occurred, little more could be done. Now, a number of treatments are available to destroy or shrink cancer that has spread to other parts of the body. Prostate cancer was one of the first forms of cancer for which these treatments were developed.

Many people expect cancer to be treated by surgical removal of all or part of the organ in which it occurs, as in cancer of the breast in women, cancer of the testis, cancer of the kidney, and many other types of cancer. Although the famous urologist Hugh Hampton Young of Johns Hopkins Hospital in Baltimore first described radical prostatectomy in 1905, the operation that removes the whole prostate gland is done on relatively few men with cancer of the prostate. The reason it is not commonly performed is that cancer of the prostate can be difficult to detect until it grows outside the prostate gland. Once this has happened, it is impossible to remove all the cancer by surgery, and an operation will not cure the disease.

Although doctors can now diagnose cancers at an earlier stage, many small early cancers grow very slowly and can take as long as 10 years to cause trouble. For a man 85 years old, this sort of tumor is not likely to be dangerous, and at this age, major surgery is usually not advisable. Removing the prostate as a treatment for cancer is done more often in younger patients or in cases in which the cancer may grow fairly quickly. Usually, the operation is recommended for men under 70, although the exact age depends on an individual's state of health.

Many prostate tumors are not immediately dangerous, and some patients may not need immediate treatment. Such patients must be tested regularly, however, in order to check that the cancer is not advancing. If the cancer grows, treatment may then be recommended. Sometimes, however, tests indicate that a tumor is growing so slowly that the patient may be advised merely to continue periodic reevaluation.

The alternative of radiation therapy can destroy small tumors and achieve cure rates similar to those of radical prostatectomy. Radiation therapy is used when the patient is not a good candidate for surgery or chooses it in preference to surgery. Although removing a tumor completely in an operation may seem more satisfactory, there is no definite proof that one method is better than the other.

Radiation therapy can also be used when surgery is not desirable because the cancer has spread outside the prostate. Here the procedure may not "cure" the cancer, but it will shrink the tumor, thereby preventing the development of further symptoms and possibly limiting its further spread.

If treatment is recommended for early-stage cancer that is confined to the prostate gland, the doctor and patient will discuss possible treatments. The best treatment for early cancer of the prostate is uncertain. A man with the disease should be informed about all of the options and actively participate in decision-making.

CHOICE OF TREATMENT

Both radical prostatectomy and radiation therapy are major treatments with potentially serious side effects. In terms of risks, overall discomfort, and time spent away from normal activities, the two treatments are not very different.

In addition, because their relative effectiveness as treatments is similar, a man with prostate cancer should be informed about the alternatives and involved in the choice of his treatment.

Some men are happier if the tumor is removed and therefore prefer surgery. Others do not like the idea of having an operation and choose radiation therapy. Surgery may not be safe for someone with severe heart or lung disease. Radiation therapy may be advised, or his condition may just be monitored (see p.63).

PRELIMINARY HORMONE TREATMENT

Sometimes, before radical prostatectomy or radiation therapy, a course of hormone treatment (see pp.67–71) is given to reduce the size of the prostate. This is thought to improve the effectiveness of the treatment and is more often done before radiation therapy treatment than before radical prostatectomy. The three-month course of hormone treatment is often associated with side effects. Once the radiation therapy or the operation has been completed, hormone treatment is stopped and its side effects should disappear. If the tumor in the prostate is particularly large, a combination of radiation therapy and continuing hormone treatment may be recommended.

RADICAL PROSTATECTOMY

Radical prostatectomy involves removal of the entire prostate gland. This is different from operations for BPH, which take out at most the inner enlarged part of the gland (see p.12). The prostate can be removed either through an incision in the lower abdomen or from below by an incision in front of the anus. Either before or at the same time, possibly by a laparoscopic "keyhole" operation, the lymph nodes at the side of the prostate will be removed and checked for signs of the cancer having spread. Removal of these nodes causes no harm. If there is no cancer in them, the only treatment needed will be the removal of the prostate gland. The process involves cutting the urethra below the prostate and removing the prostate from the neck of the bladder, which is then stitched back onto the urethra. A catheter is left in place, usually for two weeks, during the healing process. Most men get over the immediate effects of the operation quickly enough to go home after a few days with the catheter in and return to the hospital later to have it removed.

WHAT ARE THE COMPLICATIONS?

The biggest problem during the operation is a risk of bleeding from the large veins that lie in front of the prostate. A blood transfusion may be necessary if this happens. A little urine may leak from where the bladder is stitched to the urethra, but this usually stops within several days and is controlled by drains that are placed adjacent to the incision. The two problems that may occur afterward are poor control of urination and sexual difficulties.

• **Poor control of urination** The close proximity of the muscle sphincters of the bladder to the prostate was described on page 11. Removing the prostate can affect these muscles. Men commonly have some difficulty controlling the flow of urine for a day or two after the catheter is removed.

The patient is taught exercises to strengthen his muscles. Although most men regain control very quickly, some are left with a little occasional leakage during exercise or while in bed at night and may wear a pad for protection. The leakage of urine is rarely more serious. If treatment is needed, a plastic device called an artificial sphincter may be inserted in another operation.

- **Sexual problems** The nerves involved in penile erection are located close to the prostate. At one time, a radical prostatectomy almost inevitably caused a loss of erectile function because these nerves were cut. Surgeons now know the location of the nerves more precisely, and surgery is performed to avoid damage if possible. However, the surgeon will warn the patient that cutting these nerves is still sometimes necessary to remove the cancer completely. Failure of erections can usually be treated by injections into the penis. Unfortunately, the new impotence drug, sildenafil, often does not work after a radical prostatectomy in which both nerve bundles have been severed.

Nerves are easily bruised but can recover. Thus an initial loss of erection may improve but can take many months. Only erectile function is affected. Normal sexual desire and ability to reach orgasm should not be affected; however, there will be little in the way of ejaculate.

RADIATION THERAPY

When radiation therapy is administered, the patient lies under a machine for a few minutes for each treatment. A number of daily treatments, which are called "fractions," are usually given over 4–6 weeks. People normally have radiation therapy as outpatients; however, in some cases, admission to a hospital is advised.

The period of time required for radiation therapy and recuperation is comparable to the time needed in radical prostatectomy. Both treatments require a couple of months off work.

WHAT ARE THE COMPLICATIONS?

It is unusual for radiation therapy treatment to cause urinary incontinence. Failure of erection occurs quite often but less commonly than after radical prostatectomy.

Unfortunately, radiation therapy cannot be focused entirely on the prostate and consequently temporarily affects the bladder and rectum. Most men develop urinary frequency and burning as well as diarrhea during and after radiation therapy. Sometimes blood appears in the urine or bowel movements. These symptoms usually clear up within a few weeks of completion of treatment. Occasionally, symptoms persist, and, very rarely, radiation therapy may produce some permanent damage to the bladder or bowel.

An alternative way of giving radiation therapy is by surgical insertion of small radioactive "seeds" into the prostate. Interest in this method, called brachytherapy, is increasing due to improvements in the technique. However, patients have to be very carefully chosen. Only certain cancers, primarily those that are less aggressive and potentially curable, are amenable to this therapy. The patient must be able to withstand the surgery in order to implant the seeds.

TREATMENT OF ADVANCED CANCER

Unfortunately, in some cases, cancer may be too advanced to be permanently cured with surgery or radiation therapy. In others, cancer may recur after initially successful treatment with surgery. Fortunately, this is not a hopeless situation. In some cases, the tumor may grow slowly and not affect the life expectancy of an elderly man. Even when prostate cancer is more active, much can be done to relieve symptoms and slow the growth.

In addition to the usual prostatic symptoms, advanced prostate cancer most commonly causes backache and sometimes pain in other bones. It can cause general ill health, with loss of weight, anemia, and other problems. Weakening of the bones, although uncommon, can result in fractures. Occasionally, cancer in the prostate blocks the drainage of the kidneys. Often, these problems are almost completely alleviated by treatment.

Just over 50 years ago, an American urologist named Charles Huggins found that if he removed the testes from dogs with prostate cancer, their cancer shrank or regressed. He then treated some men with the same type of operation and others with female hormones. He found that their disease responded in the same way with both kinds of treatment. This was one of the earliest examples of an effective treatment for prostate cancer that had spread and was no longer amenable to surgical cure. It was so significant that Huggins was awarded the Nobel Prize for medicine. Hormone treatment is still the most effective way of treating advanced cancer of the prostate, although there are now new methods.

The prostate grows and functions only when receiving normal amounts of male hormones (androgens). There are a number of different androgens, and the most important is testosterone. Cancer of the prostate cannot grow without androgens being present. Depriving the prostate of these hormones causes the tumor to shrink and sometimes to disappear. Testosterone is produced by the testes in response to a hormone that comes from the pituitary, a small gland located at the base of the brain.

As doctors and scientists have come to understand hormones, new methods of hormone treatment have been developed. We now have more of a choice than Dr. Huggins had in the 1940s. The testes can be prevented from producing testosterone by drugs or they can be removed by an operation called an orchiectomy. Alternatively, there are drugs that act as a barrier between the tumor and the male hormones. These drugs prevent the androgens from stimulating the tumor cells without reducing the amount of androgens in the blood.

Generally speaking, the effect of these different treatments on the tumor is the same. The choice among different treatments is made on the basis of how they are administered, possible side effects, and suitability for the individual patient.

As with deciding between surgery and radiation therapy for early cancer, the patient may be asked his opinion and should have information about the possibilities. The patient can have:

- An operation, targeted at hormone production, that eliminates the need for ongoing treatment.
- A hormone injection either once a month or every third month.
- Antiandrogen drugs.

Since the hormone or drug treatments work only during the course of treatment, injections or pills must be taken indefinitely.

SURGERY AND HORMONE INJECTIONS

The usual operation to reduce male hormone levels is called a simple orchiectomy and involves removal of both of the testes. Hormone injections involve drugs called luteinizing hormone-releasing hormone (LHRH) analogues and include goserelin and leuprolide. These injections stop the production of testosterone and have effects very similar to those of the orchiectomy. Goserelin and leuprolide are now available in the form of injections and are given only once every three months. Other three-monthly hormone injections are being developed.

Whether the treatment is an operation or a hormone injection, the level of male hormones is reduced. Most men find that their sexual activity, both their desire for sex and their ability to have an erection, is consequently affected. Occasionally, for reasons that are not understood, these effects on sexual activity do not happen. Retaining sexual function does not mean that the treatment is not effective.

Hot flashes very similar to those experienced bywomen after menopause are another problem. These consist of episodes of intense heat or attacks of sweating. Most men are only mildly affected, and the condition tends to improve with the passage of time. If hot flashes are more severe, treatment is available. Hot flashes are a side effect of the treatment and not a sign that the cancer is advancing.

Surgery involves removing the testes, and the injection treatment causes the testes to shrink. Since the testes are associated with masculinity, it is therefore natural to feel that this type of treatment is "castration." However, most men with advanced prostate cancer feel so much better as the treatment starts to work that this does not usually worry them too much.

Although the operation and the injections have very similar effects in the long run, there are differences between them at the start of treatment. Orchiectomy is a fairly minor operation, but it does require hospitalization and general anesthesia. This operation also causes pain for several days after surgery. Minor complications such as bruising, swelling, and wound infection are not unusual. The operation is effective immediately. Sometimes the symptoms improve as soon as the patient wakes up after surgery.

The injections work more slowly and, during the first few weeks of treatment, they can actually cause an increase in the size of the tumor metastases, increasing the risk of pain and spinal compression fractures. An additional antiandrogen hormone (see below), such as flutamide, given orally just before and during the early phases of treatment, can be effective in preventing these effects.

OTHER DRUGS

Other antiandrogen drugs are available if the patient wants to avoid hormonal therapy and loss of sexual function. They prevent the action of testosterone on the tumor without reducing the level of testosterone in the blood. The antiandrogen medications currently available are flutamide and nilutamide. Unfortunately, these drugs tend to have side effects, including gastrointestinal upset. A new drug, bicalutamide, may have fewer side effects than either flutamide or nilutamide, but it can be used only in combination with other drugs (see p.73).

How Hormones Work

The growth of both the prostate gland and prostate cancer is controlled by the male sex hormone testosterone, made in the testes.

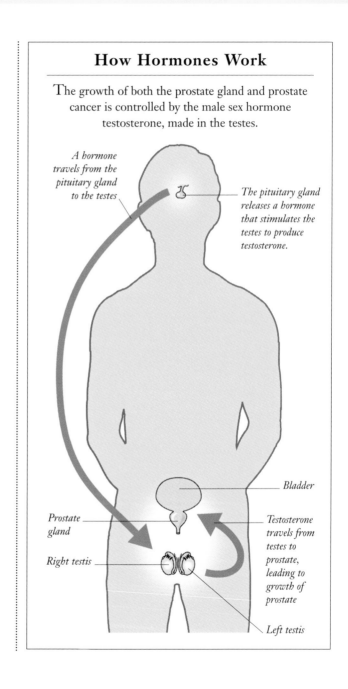

A hormone travels from the pituitary gland to the testes

The pituitary gland releases a hormone that stimulates the testes to produce testosterone.

Bladder

Prostate gland

Right testis

Testosterone travels from testes to prostate, leading to growth of prostate

Left testis

At one time, estrogen hormones were often used to treat prostate cancer. However, these hormones caused swelling of the breasts. More important, they can have serious effects on the heart. Although female hormones can be used safely in very small doses, most men are treated with one of the other types of drugs.

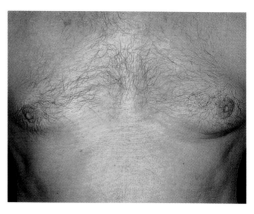

SWOLLEN BREASTS
One of the side effects of female estrogen treatment for prostate cancer is swollen breasts. This treatment is no longer prescribed in large doses.

There are other ways of giving hormone treatment, and newer and possibly better ones are always being developed. The treatments mentioned is this book are the ones most commonly used in the US.

Recently, a greater reduction of male hormone has been achieved by using a combination of drugs. The combination works because the adrenal glands also make male hormones and are not affected by orchiectomy or by using only LHRH analogues. Whether this more intensive treatment actually enhances results is still unclear. There is evidence that it does, at least in some cases, and some patients are now receiving it. Unfortunately, combination therapy is more complicated, more expensive, and can cause more side effects.

OTHER TREATMENTS

If the cancer has already spread to bone and causes pain, radiation therapy can be very effective and usually works quickly. A course of about 10 treatments is given on an outpatient or inpatient basis. Sometimes only a single treatment is necessary. Usually there are few problems, but, depending on where the painful area is, mild stomach or bowel upset might occur.

A new method of giving radiation therapy to bone uses a radioactive substance called strontium-89. This therapy selects the parts of the bone that are affected by cancer and provides very intense but localized and safe radiation. The therapy is given by injection on an outpatient basis. Some simple precautions about radiation must be followed for a day or two after the administration of the radioactive material. Strontium-89 is completely different from strontium-90, a component of radioactive fallout, and it does not have the same harmful effects.

KEY POINTS

- Prostate cancer can be treated with surgery, radiation therapy, or hormone or drug therapy.
- Removing the entire prostate, or radical prostatectomy, is effective only when the cancer is confined to the prostate.
- Radiation therapy is an alternative to radical prostatectomy and can be used to treat a tumor too advanced for surgery.
- Hormone treatment has proved useful for advanced prostate cancer.

Prostatitis

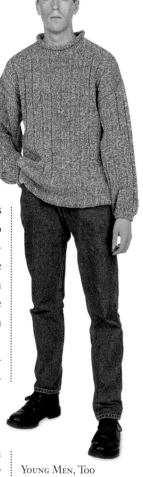

Prostatitis, or inflammation of the prostate, is generally the result of a urinary tract infection that has spread to the prostate. It is usually treated with antibiotics.

ACUTE PROSTATITIS

Inflammation of the prostate gland can occur at almost any age and is often due to infection. Although cystitis, an infection of the bladder that causes burning and frequency, more commonly affects women, these symptoms can also occur in men who develop an infection of the prostate called acute prostatitis. This condition may cause a high temperature and make the patient feel very sick. In an older man who also has BPH, prostate symptoms might become worse, and prostatitis can sometimes result in retention of urine.

Sometimes an infection of the testes called epididymitis complicates prostatitis, and the resulting symptoms can overshadow those from the prostate. Like simple cystitis, epididymitis is treated with antibiotics. However, many antibiotics do not penetrate very well and may not be effective. If an infection of the prostate is suspected, the antibiotic most likely to be used is one from the quinolone group, which includes ciprofloxacin, ofloxacin, levofloxacin, and norfloxacin. The antibiotic must be taken long enough to

YOUNG MEN, TOO
Infection of the prostate can affect men of all ages and can cause symptoms similar to those of cystitis.

75

eradicate the infection completely. This usually requires several weeks of treatment. The full course of antibiotics must be taken, even if the symptoms have disappeared, to prevent the infection from recurring.

Drink plenty of fluids, rest, and avoid intercourse when you feel ill. Most patients will not be interested in sexual activity while the symptoms are bad. Afterward, however, frequent sexual activity might be helpful because every time a climax is reached, the fluid from the prostate gland may flush out any remaining infection. In rare instances, an abscess develops. This is treated by letting out the pus by an operation very similar to a TURP.

CHRONIC PROSTATITIS

This condition can lead to occasional flare-ups of cystitis-like symptoms or cause more chronic pain. Such pain occurs in the lower abdomen, the testes, between the legs, or even in the rectal area. Chronic prostatitis can be very difficult to diagnose. Its symptoms can be caused by all sorts of conditions that do not necessarily involve the prostate. If symptoms are caused by prostatitis, the prostate may be tender on examination. The doctor may try to grow bacteria from the prostatic fluid, which can be obtained by massaging the prostate, or from semen.

MAKING A DIAGNOSIS
Culturing a sample of fluid from the prostate for bacteria will confirm a diagnosis of prostatitis.

Sometimes the prostate gland is inflamed but does not seem to be infected by bacteria. The cause of this type of prostatitis is not really understood, but the symptoms are sometimes helped by anti-inflammatory drugs such as ibuprofen and indomethacin.

PROSTATODYNIA

Symptoms similar to those of prostatitis are caused by a condition called prostatodynia, which probably results from spasm of the muscle in the prostate gland. Many men who suffer from prostatodynia are helped by the alpha-blocker drugs that are used for BPH (see pp.45–46).

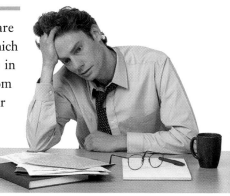

Conditions caused by muscle spasm are often aggravated by anxiety and stress. Symptoms are likely to occur during a difficult time at work. Worrying about the condition can also make it worse. In such cases, it is wise to have the prostate checked and receive assurance that nothing else is wrong. Pain in the prostate is rarely caused by cancer, but unexplained symptoms should always be further investigated.

STRESSED OUT
Anxiety and stress can bring on the muscle spasms that cause prostatodynia.

KEY POINTS

- Inflammation of the prostate, or prostatitis, may be caused by infection.
- Treatment is usually with antibiotics.

Improving treatment

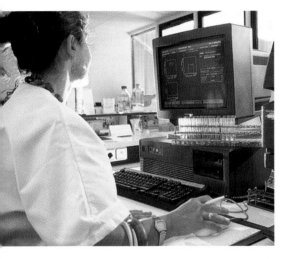

Although there have been many new developments in managing prostate disorders, finding a way to prevent common disorders like BPH would be a major step forward in improving men's health.

Preventing BPH may already be possible. The new prostate drug finasteride may be better at preventing BPH than at treating the condition once it exists. Unfortunately, all men would have to start taking the drug at age 40 and continue every day for the rest of their lives. Since the condition in most cases is a nuisance rather than life-threatening, this is not practical.

As new, more effective drugs are found and technologies such as thermotherapy and laser devices are improved, the day may come when TURP and other "old-fashioned" prostate operations are no longer done.

Cancer of the prostate is a far too common disease. If treatments were simpler and easier than the current ones – prostate removal and radiation therapy – screening for early disease might be more cost-effective. We are beginning to learn more about the causes of prostate cancer and are continually seeking ways of preventing it. Trials of drugs that stop the development of cancer of the prostate are under way.

CLINICAL TRIALS

Many new methods of treatment for both BPH and cancer are under investigation. Such treatments can be tested only with the help of people who have the disease. Their participation in clinical trials is an essential part of evaluating the safety and effectiveness of new treatments.

If you have a prostate condition, you might be asked to take part in a clinical trial. Usually, this will be before treatment with drugs that have already been extensively tested and are therefore almost certainly safe. Being in a clinical trial is some-times the only way to be treated with a promising new drug.

Most clinical trials are double-blind, randomized studies. These either compare two different drug treatments or compare one treatment against an inactive, or "dummy," medication known as a placebo. The compari-son is worthwhile only if the treatment that each patient is given is chosen

HELPING IN TRIALS
In clinical trials, you may either be given an active treatment or a placebo. Neither you nor the doctor will know which you are given.

by chance, or randomized. To interpret the results fairly, neither the patients nor the doctors running the trial know which medications each patient is taking. However, if a patient really needs to know, the type of treatment can easily be determined.

WHY IS A PLACEBO NECESSARY?

Simply seeing a doctor tends to make you feel better. This is known as the placebo effect and is frequently seen in trials of BPH treatments. It may occur because the attention makes patients less concerned about their disease, resulting in relaxation of the muscle in the prostate. Patients receiving the placebo treatment may therefore notice fewer symptoms, and their flow rate may also improve. It is very important to compare active drugs to a placebo to make sure that the drug, not some other factor, is the cause of the improvement.

If you do take part in a clinical trial, you will receive a lot of attention, which many patients appreciate. On the other hand, you must visit the doctor more often, and some people find this difficult. The main disadvantage in most trials is the need for many blood samples. If you cannot tolerate frequent testing, participation in a trial may not be appropriate for you.

Before a clinical trial is allowed to take place, the Food and Drug Administration must endorse it as reasonably safe and sensible. You should be given a full explanation of the trial both orally by a doctor and in writing. It is entirely your choice whether you take part. You should not take part simply to please the doctor. No one will object if you do not accept an invitation to participate in a clinical trial. You will still get all necessary approved treatment. However, most patients who take part in trials usually enjoy the process and benefit from the treatment.

WHO WILL TREAT YOU?

Many diseases are treated by both specialists and primary care physicians, sometimes jointly. Patients with diabetes and high blood pressure are familiar with this. Until recently, the only real treatment for BPH, the most common disease of the prostate, was an operation. Unless the primary care physician decided that the problem was so mild that no treatment was needed, a referral to a urologist was obviously the best thing for the patient. Even now, many men who have prostate problems are seen and evaluated by a urologist.

However, the treatment of prostate disorders has changed because of the availability of drugs for BPH. Men with prostate symptoms are now less tolerant of their symptoms. People are living longer; consequently, more men are old enough to have prostate trouble than in the past.

Since milder forms of BPH can be managed with drugs, it is no longer absolutely necessary for a urologist to treat every patient. However, it is important that the patient be carefully evaluated before starting treatment to make sure that drugs are the correct choice and to rule out cancer or other serious conditions that need to be treated by a urologist.

KEY POINTS

- Determined efforts are under way to find better treatments for prostate disorders.
- Clinical trials are essential to show that a treatment really works and is safe.

Case histories

Case History 1: **PROSTATE CANCER**

Alan James, a man of 68, had a transurethral resection of the prostate (TURP) for benign prostatic hyperplasia (BPH) a few years ago, but he developed recurrent symptoms of dribbling and frequent urination. When he was examined, his prostate was small but very hard, and some excised tissue showed cancer. Radiation therapy of the prostate was planned, but a bone scan showed that there were a few small areas of cancer in the spine. Since these were causing no symptoms, he decided not to be treated. However, he knew the importance of close monitoring and was seen by the urologist every few months and had his PSA level measured. Over the next 15 months, his PSA slowly started to rise and prostate symptoms returned. Although his bone scan had not altered, he agreed to have hormone treatment. Not wanting to lose his potency, Mr. James was treated with flutamide. His prostate symptoms improved, and within three months, the PSA had become completely normal. He remained well for 18 months, when the PSA started to rise again. He was started on injections of an LHRH drug, and then the flutamide was stopped. He remains well, and his PSA has fallen again.

This tells us a lot about cancer of the prostate. Since cancer develops in the outer part of the prostate, having a TURP for BPH does not mean that cancer cannot develop later. When the disease is detected at a fairly early stage, a delay in treatment may not matter. The risk of side effects is reduced by delaying treatment and by choosing the right treatment for the patient, in this case flutamide because Mr. James wanted to remain potent. Although the beneficial effect of hormone treatment may not be permanent, changing treatment, as in this case, is sometimes helpful. Mr. James has been fortunate and has been well for several years. His case illustrates that cancer of the prostate, even when it cannot be cured, can often be kept under control. Since effective treatment options are available, it is important to keep patient appointments, especially if treatment has been deferred. Note the amount of choice and control Mr. James had over his treatment.

Case History 2: RETENTION OF URINE

Robert Cohen, aged 90, consulted a urologist because he was having trouble urinating. The urologist found that his prostate was quite large. Mr. Cohen's PSA measured almost 10 times the normal level, suggesting that cancer of the prostate was likely. Mr. Cohen's advanced age and poor health made it difficult to determine the best treatment. In the meantime, he was admitted to the hospital because he was retaining urine and needed a catheter. He could not urinate when the catheter was removed and therefore needed an operation. Since the prostate was so large, an open procedure was required. The prostate weighed more than 12 ounces (350 g), six times more than most enlarged prostates. The pathology examination revealed BPH with no evidence of cancer.

An open operation, although somewhat old-fashioned, is still the best way to deal with a very large prostate. In BPH, the level of PSA depends on the size of the gland. If the gland is unusually large or if the patient has cancer, the PSA is also much higher than would be expected with BPH. This emphasizes the problems of using PSA to diagnose cancer.

Case History 3: **BLADDER TUMOR**

Ray Phillips, age 60, was admitted to the hospital for an elective prostate resection, or partial removal. Two days before he entered the hospital, he noticed blood in his urine for the first time. Although the bleeding had stopped, the urologist did a careful cystoscopy examination of the bladder before starting the TURP and found a small tumor in the lining of the bladder that was simple to remove at the same time.

It is never safe to assume that bleeding is from the prostate, even if the prostate is causing other symptoms. If another cause is found, it is most often a bladder tumor. Although there is no connection between bladder tumors and BPH, men with bladder tumors commonly have BPH as well.

Case History 4: **URETHRAL STRICTURE**

Sam Goldstein, a man of 65, complained of difficulty urinating about six months after a coronary artery bypass graft performed for angina. His prostate was enlarged, and he was referred to a urologist to determine whether a prostate operation was needed. The urologist did a cystoscopy and found a stricture in the urethra. The stricture was cut open by a small operation called a urethrotomy, performed with an instrument similar to that used to do a TURP. This completely cured Mr. Goldstein's symptoms even though his prostate was enlarged.

Other disorders can cause symptoms commonly seen in prostate disease, and an enlarged prostate itself may not be the cause of trouble. A catheter is used during heart operations to assist the flow of urine. The urologist knew that this can occasionally cause a urethral stricture and recommended a cystoscopic examination.

Case History 5: SUBMEATAL STRICTURE

Two months after a TURP, Andrew Roberts felt that his symptoms were coming back and noticed that his urine was spraying out of his penis. He went back to the urologist, who performed cystoscopy and diagnosed a short stricture just behind the external urinary opening. The stricture was gently stretched with metal dilators. After this had been done a few times, Mr. Roberts had no more trouble.

A submeatal stricture is not unusual after a TURP and is easily treated. Do not despair if all is not going completely smoothly after a prostate operation. Many of the problems are easy to correct.

Case History 6: ELEVATED PSA

Having had mild prostate symptoms for a few years, 70-year-old John Pearson saw his doctor because the symptoms had suddenly become worse. A blood test showed that Mr. Pearson's PSA was significantly elevated. Although the PSA was not very high, it suggested the possibility of cancer. He saw a urologist shortly thereafter. The urologist examined the prostate, which felt benign, and retested the PSA, which was now lower. This was reassuring. Two months later, the PSA had returned to normal and Mr. Pearson's symptoms had disappeared. Nothing more had to be done.

Mr. Pearson clearly had some sudden event affecting his prostate, perhaps a mild infection or a little internal bleeding sufficient to cause bruising or swelling without blood appearing in the urine. Sometimes an enlarged prostate can lose part of its blood supply, and the "dead" area causes temporary swelling. Some urologists believe that this happens to men who suddenly get retention when they have had no previous trouble. When something like this happens, a greater amount of PSA is released into the blood and the elevated level is detected by the blood test. A single PSA measurement is not conclusive and cannot be used alone to diagnose cancer. In fact, BPH might have provided a better explanation for Mr. Pearson's elevated PSA level when he was first seen.

Case History 7: **ACUTE PROSTATITIS**

William Hadley, a 58-year-old man, returned from a dinner party, experienced severe and burning pain when urinating, and noticed that his urinary stream was poor. He had a sudden attack of shivering and a few hours later developed a high fever. Mr. Hadley called his doctor, who started him on antibiotics. He felt better, but continued to have difficulty urinating. When the urine flow almost completely stopped, Mr. Hadley saw a urologist, who advised immediate admission to the hospital. His prostate was firm and tender. His PSA was six times normal. A catheter was inserted, and the antibiotics were continued. After a few days, he was able to urinate when the catheter was removed, although he still had some difficulty. He continued to take antibiotics and his symptoms gradually disappeared. His PSA declined but took two months to return to normal. Once he had recovered, Mr. Hadley once again had a soft and benign prostate, but his urine flow rate was still well below normal.

Mr. Hadley had severe acute prostatitis. The fact that his flow rate upon recovery was reduced suggested that he probably already had some obstruction from his prostate. The swelling from the prostatitis and perhaps from drinking alcohol pushed him into urine retention. Acute prostatitis can make the prostate feel hard and can cause very high levels of PSA. Indeed, it may be best not to measure PSA in this situation. The high PSA takes a long time to return to normal. Mr. Hadley took antibiotics for six weeks. Stopping the treatment for prostatitis too soon can lead to relapse.

Questions and answers

Why do benign prostatic hyperplasia (BPH) and cancer of the prostate occur only in older men?

Some growth of the prostate probably occurs throughout adult life under the influence of male hormones. Around the age of 50, changes take place in the way the body produces and deals with male hormones. This seems to cause the more rapid growth seen in BPH. These hormone changes may influence development of cancer of the prostate. However, many other types of cancer also occur more commonly in older people, probably because whatever causes the cancer takes many years to produce its effect.

Why do some men with BPH get no symptoms?

We do not quite understand this. Certainly a small hypertrophied prostate can cause very bad symptoms, while men with huge prostates can have virtually no trouble. It probably depends partly on just how the prostate squeezes the urethra and how well the bladder can cope with obstruction. There are probably very few elderly men who are not affected, but many have mild symptoms that are virtually unnoticeable.

Will having sexual intercourse frequently make me more likely to have prostatic disease?

No, but it is not protective either. A study of abstinent men showed that they were just as likely to get cancer of the prostate as sexually active men.

Can disease of the prostate cause illness in sexual partners?

No. BPH is specific to the prostate and therefore cannot occur in women. It is not caused by anything that can be sexually transmitted. The same applies to prostate cancer. Although the prostate may be affected by sexually transmitted infections, this is unusual. Prostatitis poses no risk to the patient's partner and is not sexually transmitted.

I sometimes see blood in my semen. Is this a sign of prostate disease?

Blood in the semen is quite common but not always noticed. Unlike blood in the urine, it is rarely a sign of serious illness. It can be compared to a nosebleed. Like nosebleeds, it can sometimes occur repeatedly for a short period of time and then stop. Both nosebleeds and blood in the semen are usually harmless. Very rarely, however, they can be signs of other disease or the result of some localized disease that causes bleeding. Occasionally, blood in the semen is associated with small stones in the prostate, which can sometimes complicate prostatitis. Although BPH and prostate cancer can cause bleeding, blood is usually seen in the urine. If you repeatedly notice blood in the semen, you should see your doctor.

Can I do anything to reduce the risk of prostate disease?

Probably not. However, if you have prostate trouble, keep it from getting worse by being sensible. Drink enough fluids, and spread them evenly through the day. If you are liable to wake at night, cut down your fluid intake in the evening and do not drink a lot of tea, coffee, or beer before going to bed. Avoid deferring urination and make a point of urinating regularly at comfortable intervals. On the other hand, it is easy to get into the habit of urinating more often than necessary, and this should be avoided because it not only makes things worse but also interferes with your regular activities.

I just had prostatitis. Does this mean that I am likely to get prostate trouble in old age?

Not really. Prostatitis does not cause either BPH or cancer. Of course, prostate trouble is common, and you may develop it anyway.

I sometimes have pain in my testes. Is this due to prostate disease?

Pain in the testes is a very common symptom. Usually no cause is found, and the pain goes away without treatment. The testes are normally sensitive, and sometimes this sensitivity increases for no apparent reason. Discomfort occurs from time to time in men who have had vasectomy operations. Since the tubes from the testes go into the prostate, it is possible for infection from the prostate to spread into them. Painful swelling of the epididymis, which is attached to the back of the testes, is called epididymitis and sometimes occurs in men with BPH or prostatitis. If you feel a hard lump in your testis, it could be a tumor and should be examined by your doctor immediately.

My father died from cancer of the prostate. Is the same thing likely to happen to me?

Not necessarily. However, there seems to be a type of prostate cancer that runs in families. If two or more closely related members of your family have had prostate cancer, especially when they were fairly young, have your prostate checked regularly once you turn 40, as recommended by the American Cancer Society.

I have heard that there is an herbal treatment for the prostate. Is this better than having an operation or taking drugs?

A large number of herbal treatments are said to help prostate disease, and they are gaining in popularity. In fact, the Worldwide Fund for Nature is now worried because a tree species has almost been wiped out because its bark is thought to be an effective treatment for BPH.

Most of these treatments have not been properly tested. If they seem to work, it may just be a placebo effect (see p.80). However, there is no reason why plants should not produce substances that work a bit like the drugs prescribed for BPH. One such remedy is saw palmetto, which may be effective in reducing the symptoms of BPH.

You should be aware that these plant substances could have just as many, if not more, side effects as prescription drugs do and may not be any safer. If you want to try a medication to help your prostate, you should ask your doctor about one of the drugs described on pp.44–47. They have been proven to be effective and safe.

I am just 50. If I am likely to experience prostate trouble, could I have an operation now to prevent it?

No! A transurethral resection of the prostate (TURP) is not used to prevent potential difficulties but only to treat actual problems caused by BPH. Complications such as a urethral stricture might occur and cause other, equally aggravating symptoms. In addition, you would have retrograde ejaculation for the rest of your life.

Useful addresses

American Cancer Society
Online: www.cancer.org
1599 Clifton Road, NE
Atlanta, GA 30329
Tel: (800) 586-4872

Center for Prostate Disease Research
Department of Surgery
Uniformed Services University of
Health Sciences
4301 Jones Bridge Road
Bethesda, MD 20814
Tel: (301) 295-9826

National Institute on Aging
Information Center
Online: wwww.nih.gov/nia
PO Box 8057
Gaithersburg, MD 20898
Tel: (800) 222-2225

National Kidney and Urologic
Diseases Information Clearinghouse
Online: www.niddk.nih.gov/health/
kidney/nkudic.htm
3 Information Way
Bethesda, MD 20892
Tel: (301) 654-4415

Prostate Health Council
The American Foundation for
Urologic Disease
Online: www.afud.org
1126 North Charles Street
Baltimore, MD 21201
Tel: (401) 468-1800

The Prostatitis Foundation
Online: www.prostate.org
1063 30th Street, Box 8
Smithshire, IL 61478
Tel: (888) 891-4200

Notes

Notes

Index

A

aging process 24–5
 BPH 17–8, 88
 obstruction 12–13
alpha-blocker drugs 45–7, 77
ambulatory urodynamics 35
anesthetics 40
anatomy 10–13
antiandrogens 71–3
anti-inflammatories 76
antibiotics 75–6
artificial sphincters 65

B

benign prostatic hyperplasia
 (BPH) 17–18, 34, 88–90
 case histories 84, 85
 treatment 37–49, 78–81
bicalutamide 73
biopsies 33, 54–5
bladder
 aging process 24–5
 irritative symptoms 14–15
 obstruction 12–14
 stones 17, 22, 23–4
 tumors 22, 23–4, 25, 85
 unstable 34
bleeding 17
 bladder tumors 24, 25, 85
 examinations 32–3, 35, 36
 postoperative 40–1, 42, 64
 radiation therapy 66
 semen 89
blood tests 31, 53–7
bone scan test 61, 83
BPH *see* benign prostatic
 hyperplasia
brachytherapy 66
breast swelling 73

C

cancer 8, 19–20, 58–74
 aging process 88
 case histories 83–4
 genetic susceptibility 90
 PSA 53–7
 sex 88
 treatment 62–74, 79
case histories 83–7
catheters
 BHP treatment 40–2, 48
 cancer treatment 64
 cystometrograms 34–5
 urethral strictures 22–3
 urinary retention 50–2
clinical trials 79–81
cystitis symptoms 75, 76
cystometrogram 34–5, 36
cystoscopy 25, 35–6, 86

D

diet, cancer 59
doxazosin 46
drinking 37, 89
drug treatments 44–7, 69–73,
 75–82
dysuria
 cystoscopy 36
 infections 17
 prostatitis 18, 87

E

ejaculation, retrograde
 43, 46, 90
embarrassment 7, 9, 30
epididymitis 75, 89
erections 65, 71
estrogens 73
examinations 27–36, 81

F

finasteride 45–7, 78
flutamide 72–3, 83–4
foreskin problems 30
frequency 14–15, 34

G

genetic susceptibility, prostate
 cancer 90
goserelin 70

H

Hampton Young,
 Hugh 62
heat treatment 47–8
hematuria 25, 85
 examinations 35, 36
 postoperative 40–1, 42
 radiation therapy 66
herbal treatments 90
hesitancy 13, 14
hormone treatments
 BPH 44–7, 78
 cancer 67–73, 84–5
hot flashes 71
Huggins, Charles 69
hyperthermia 47–8

I

incomplete emptying 14
incomplete sensation 15
intravenous urogram (IVU)
 25, 32–3
irritative symptoms 14–15, 24,
 37

K

kidney disorders
 failure 38, 52
 stones 33
 tumors 25

L

laser treatment 47, 48
leuprolide 70
luteinizing hormone releasing-
  hormone (LHRH)
  analogue 70, 83–4

N

nilutamide 71

O

obstruction 22–4
  examinations 31–2, 34–5
  symptoms 13–14
  treatment 38, 46–7
operations *see* surgery
orchiectomy 69–71

P

pain
  see also dysuria
  cancer 74
  prostatitis 76
  testes 89
  TURP 41
  urine retention 15, 50
phimosis 30
placebos 79–80, 90
prazosin 46
primary care physician 27, 81
prostate-specific antigen (PSA)
  31, 53–7, 83–4
  case histories 83–4, 86–7
prostatitis 18, 75–7, 89
  case histories 87
prostatodynia 77

Q

questionnaires 28–9
quinolones 75–6

R

radical prostatectomy 56–7,
  60, 63–5, 67
radiation therapy 63, 66–7, 70
  strontium-89 74
rectal examinations 30
retention of urine 15–17
  case histories 84
  treatment 38, 50–2
risk reduction 89

S

screening, cancer 55–7
semen 89
sex 88
  hormone therapy 44–5, 71,
    72
  postoperative 42, 43, 64–5
  prostatitis 76
sleep loss 14–15, 24
sphincters 11–12, 43, 65
stents 49
stress 77
strontium-89 74
submeatal stricture 86
surgery 8, 90
  BPH 37–44, 46–7
  cancer 56–7, 61–2, 63–5,
    67, 69–70
symptoms 12–17, 22–5, 37

T

tamsulosin 46
terazosin 46
testes 69–72, 76, 89
testosterone 44–5, 68, 70–3
tests 30–6, 53–7, 59–61
thermotherapy 47–8
transrectal ultrasound
  scan 33–4, 55, 61

transurethral resection of the
  prostate (TURP) 91
  BHP 38–44
  cancer 61
  case histories 85–6
tumors *see* bladder tumors;
  cancer of the prostate
TURP *see* transurethral
  resection of the prostate

U

ultrasound scans 33–4
urethra 12–13
urethral stricture 22–3, 35, 85
urgency 14, 34
urination 12–17, 24–5
  see also hematuria (blood in
    the urine)
  burning sensations 17, 18,
    36, 87
  dribbling 14, 43–4
  flow measurement 31–2,
    34–5
  irritative symptoms 13–17
  nighttime 15, 24, 43
  obstruction 13–14
  postoperative 42–4, 64–5
  retention 15–17, 38, 50–2,
    84
  samples 31
urologist 27–32, 38–41, 81

V

vaporization 48

X

X-rays 25, 32, 61

Acknowledgments

PUBLISHER'S ACKNOWLEDGMENTS
Dorling Kindersley Publishing, Inc. would like to thank the following for their help and participation in this project:

Managing Editor Stephanie Jackson; **Managing Art Editor** Nigel Duffield;
Editorial Assistance Judit Z. Bodnar, Janel Bragg, Alrica Goldstein, Mary Lindsay, Jennifer Quasha, Ashley Ren, Design Revolution;
Design Assistance Sarah Hall, Marianne Markham, Design Revolution, Chris Walker; **Production** Michelle Thomas, Elizabeth Cherry.

Consultancy Dr. Tony Smith, Dr. Sue Davidson;
Indexing Indexing Specialists, Hove; **Administration** Christopher Gordon.

Illustrations: (p.11, p.12, p.13, p.19, p.23, p.41) ©Philip Wilson; (p.72) Mark Roberts.

Picture Research: Angela Anderson, Andy Samson;
Picture Librarian: Charlotte Oster.

PICTURE CREDITS
The publisher would like to thank the following for their kind permission to reproduce their photographs. Every effort has been made to trace the copyright holders. Dorling Kindersley apologizes for any unintentional omissions and would be pleased, in any such cases, to add an acknowledgment in future editions.

APM Studios p.50; **Science Photo Library** p.20, p.22 (Michael Abbey), p.32 (CNR), p.37 (Mura Jerrican), p.54 (St. Bartholomew's Hospital), p.58 (Conor Caffrey), p.73 (Dr. P. Marazzi), p.76 (Geoff Tompkinson), p.78 (BSIP LECA).